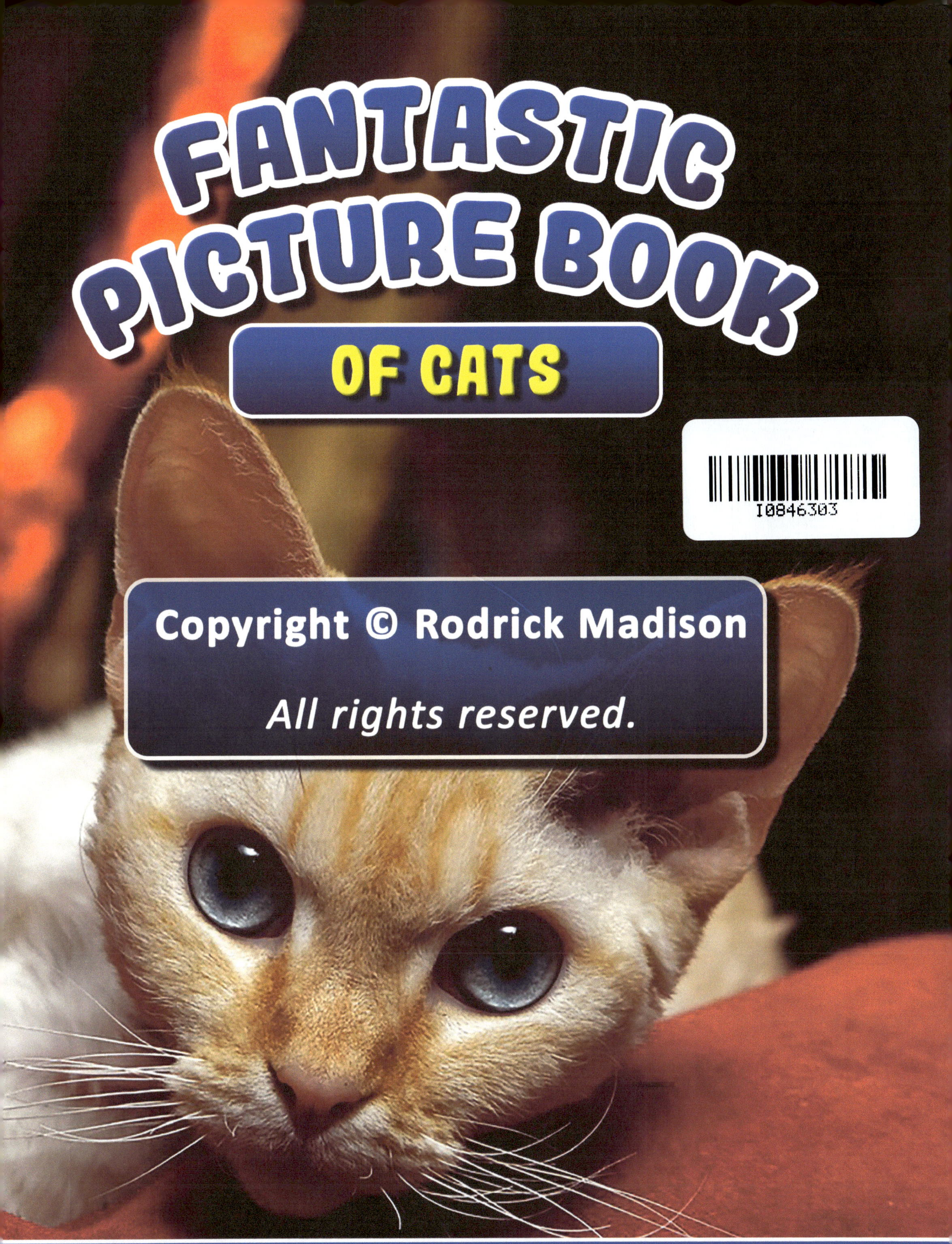

FANTASTIC PICTURE BOOK

OF CATS

Copyright © Rodrick Madison

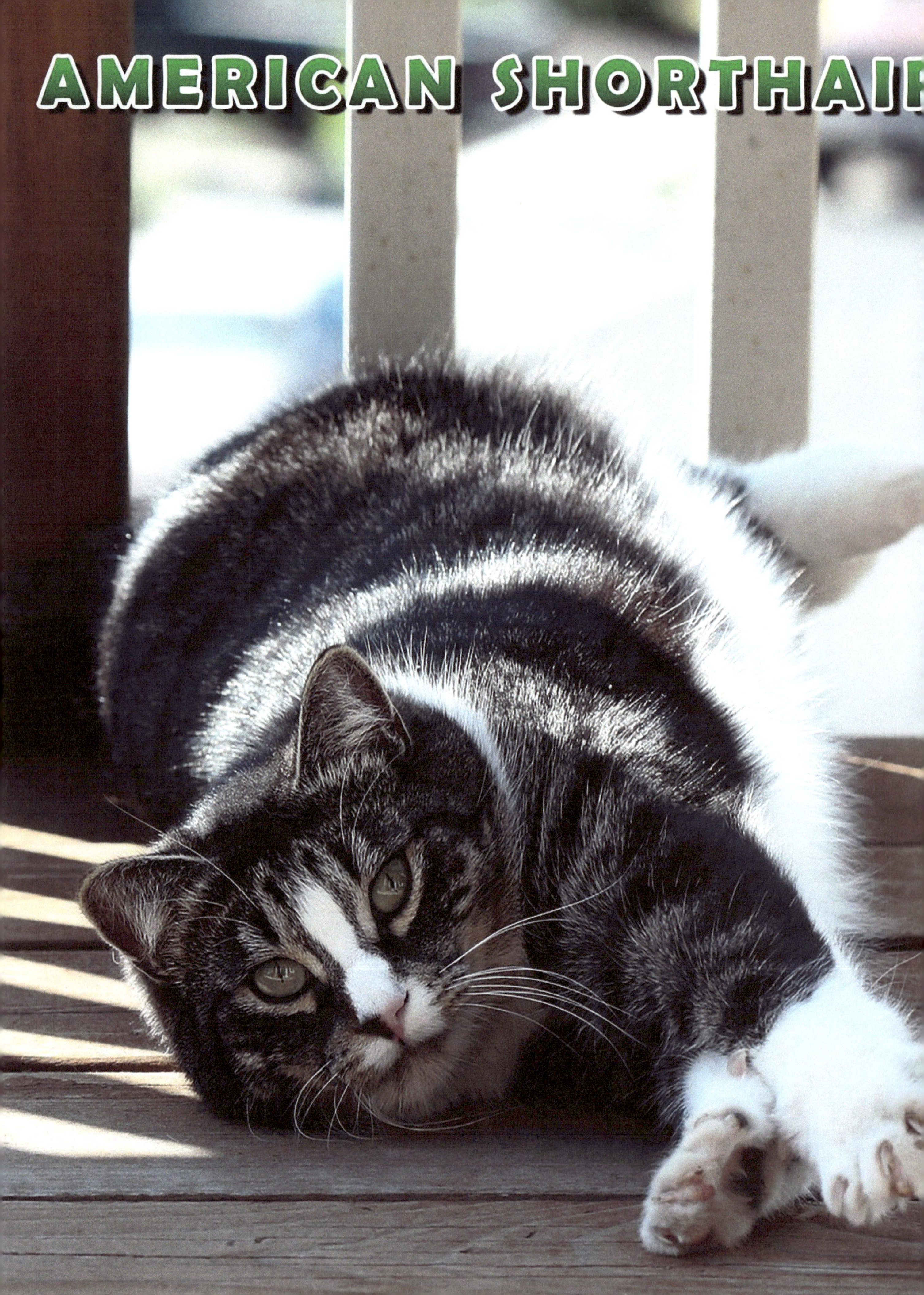

AMERICAN SHORTHAIR

ABYSSINIAN CAT

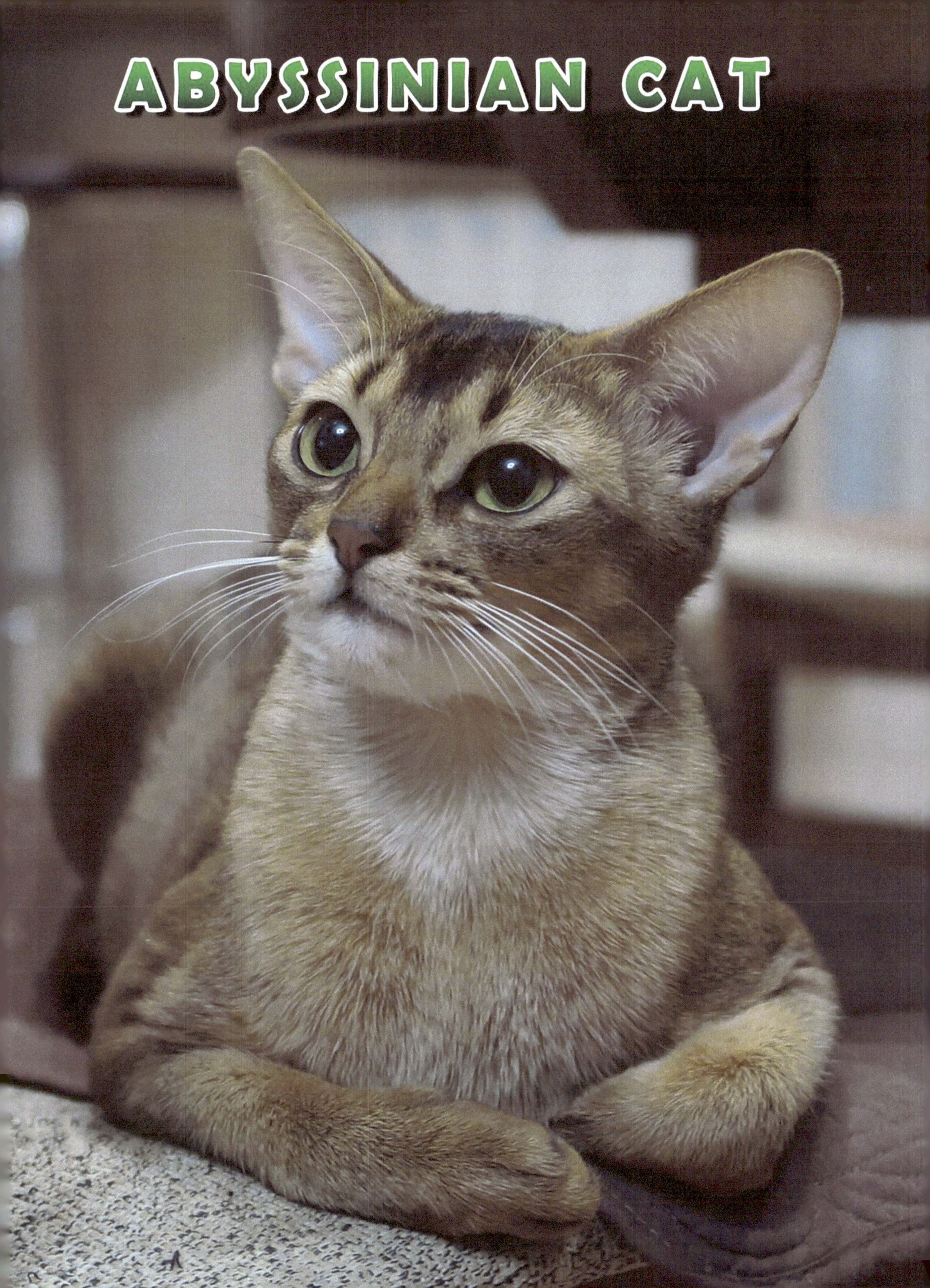

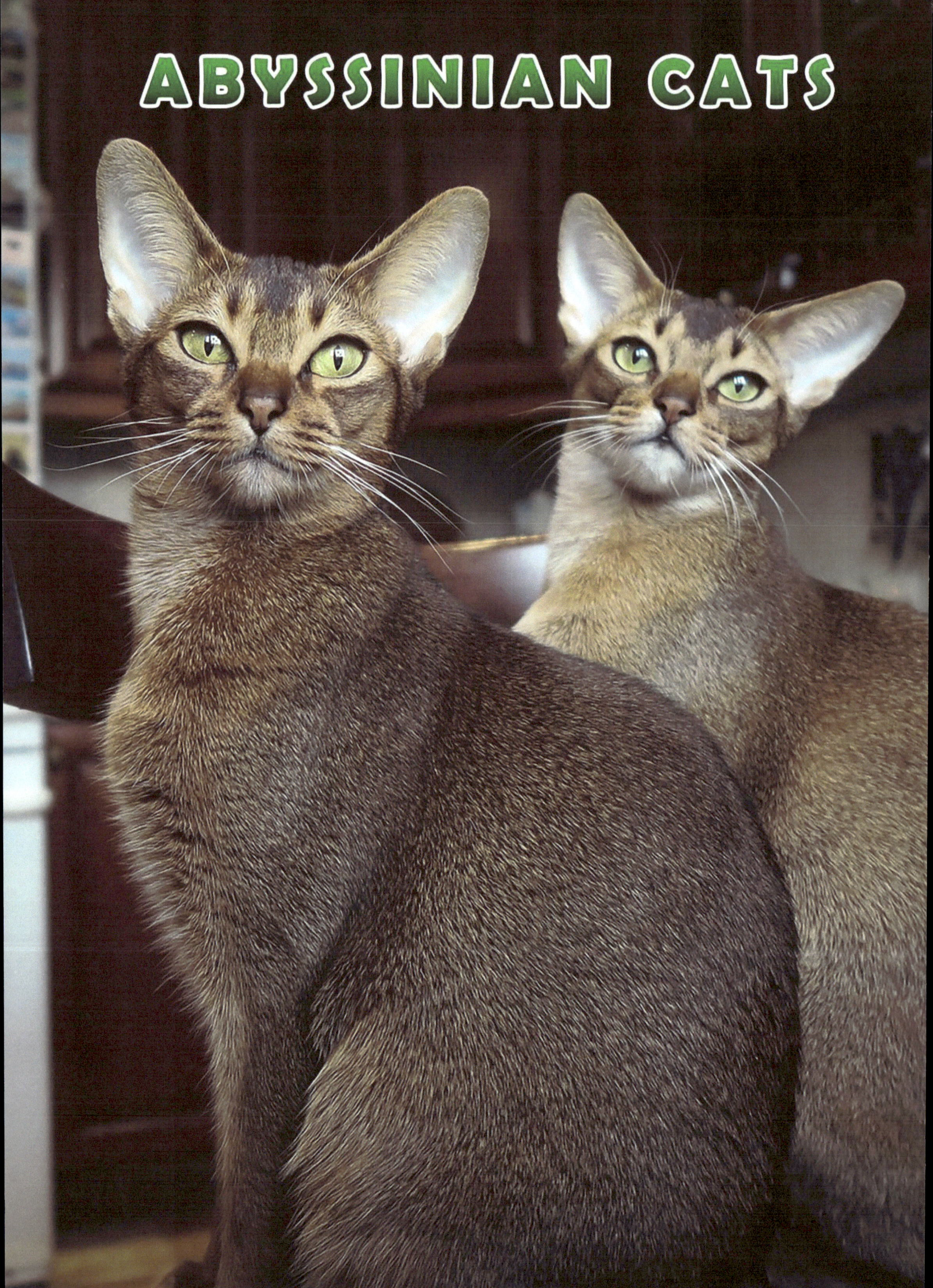
ABYSSINIAN CATS

BENGAL CAT

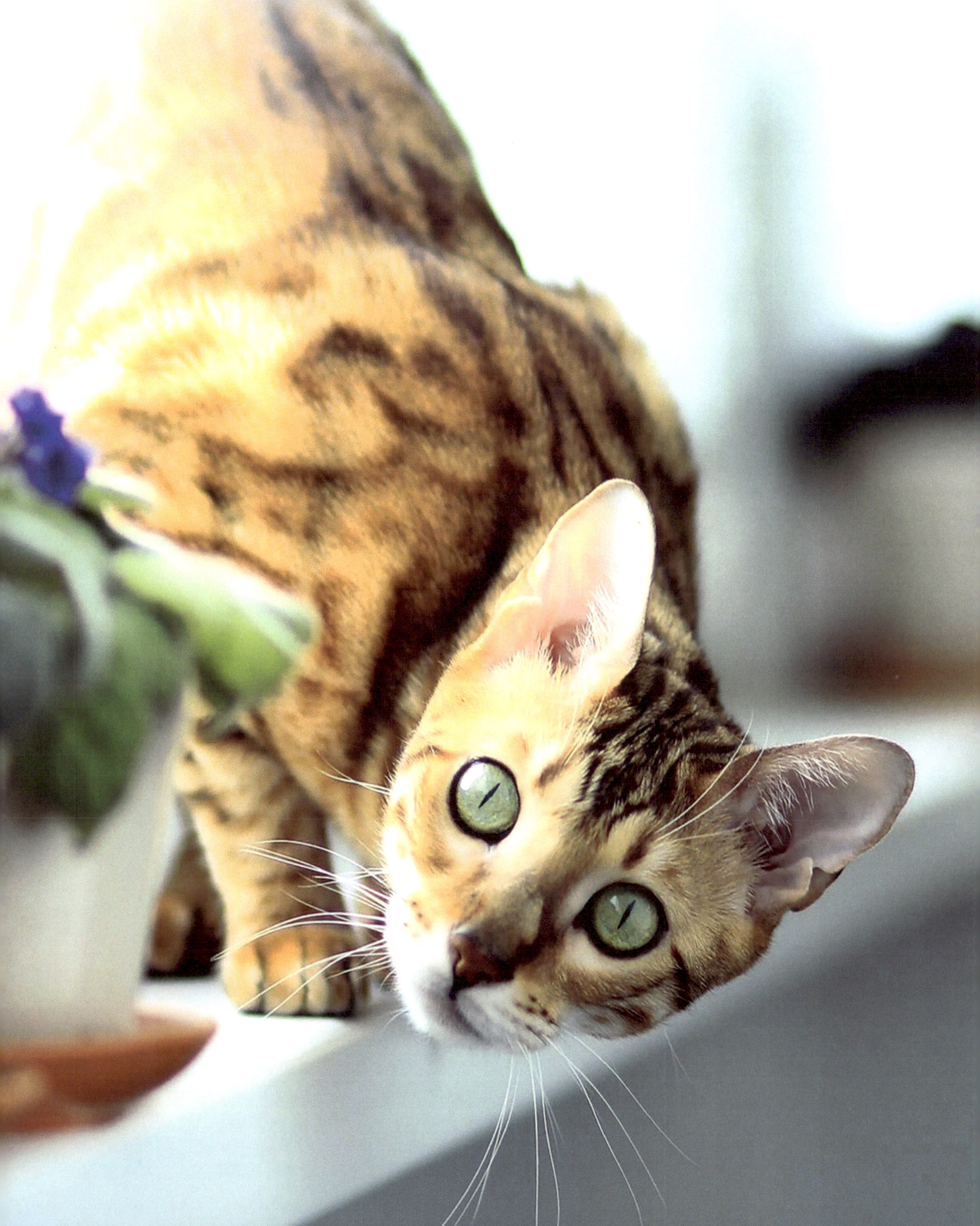

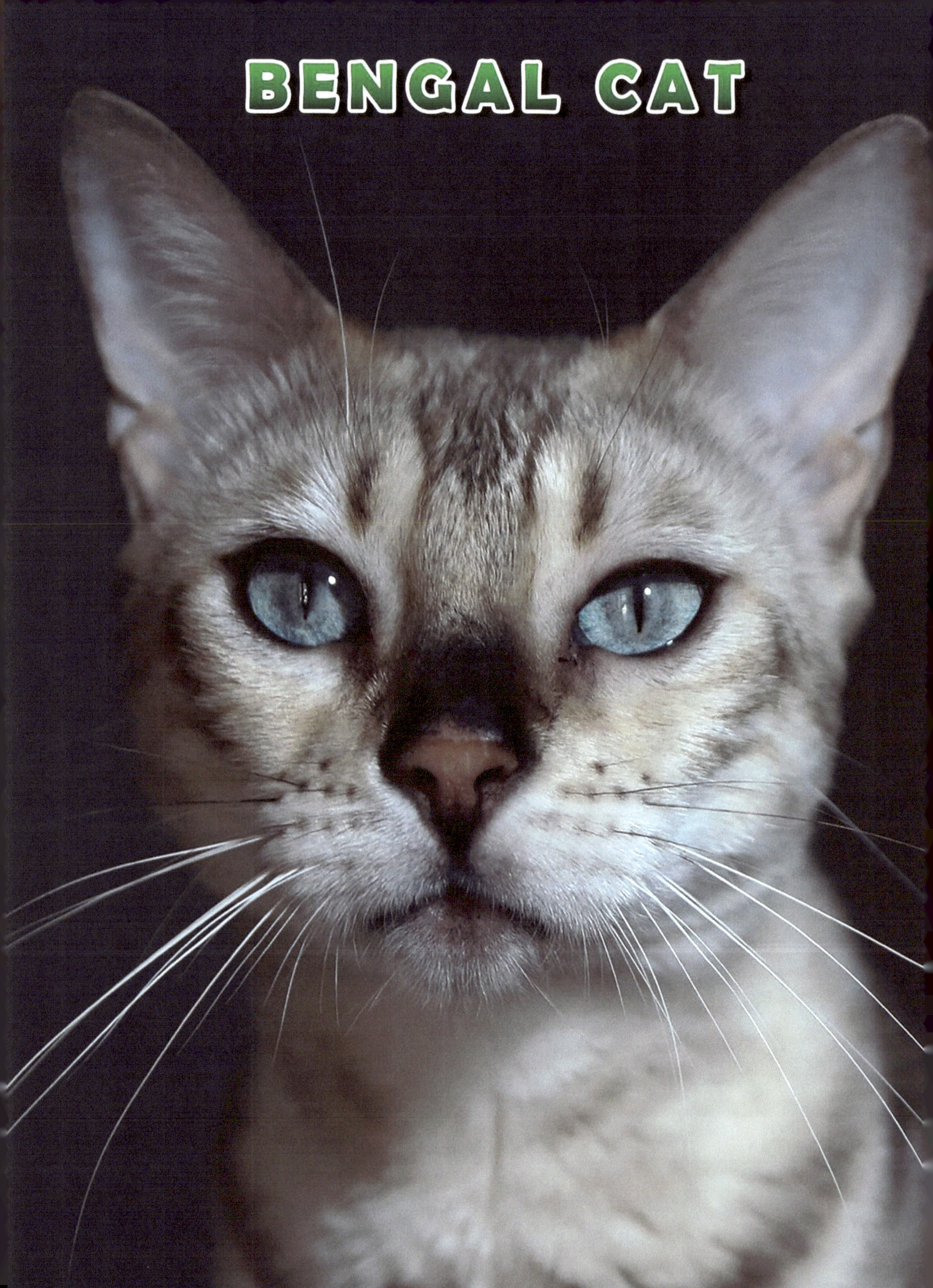
BENGAL CAT

BIRMAN

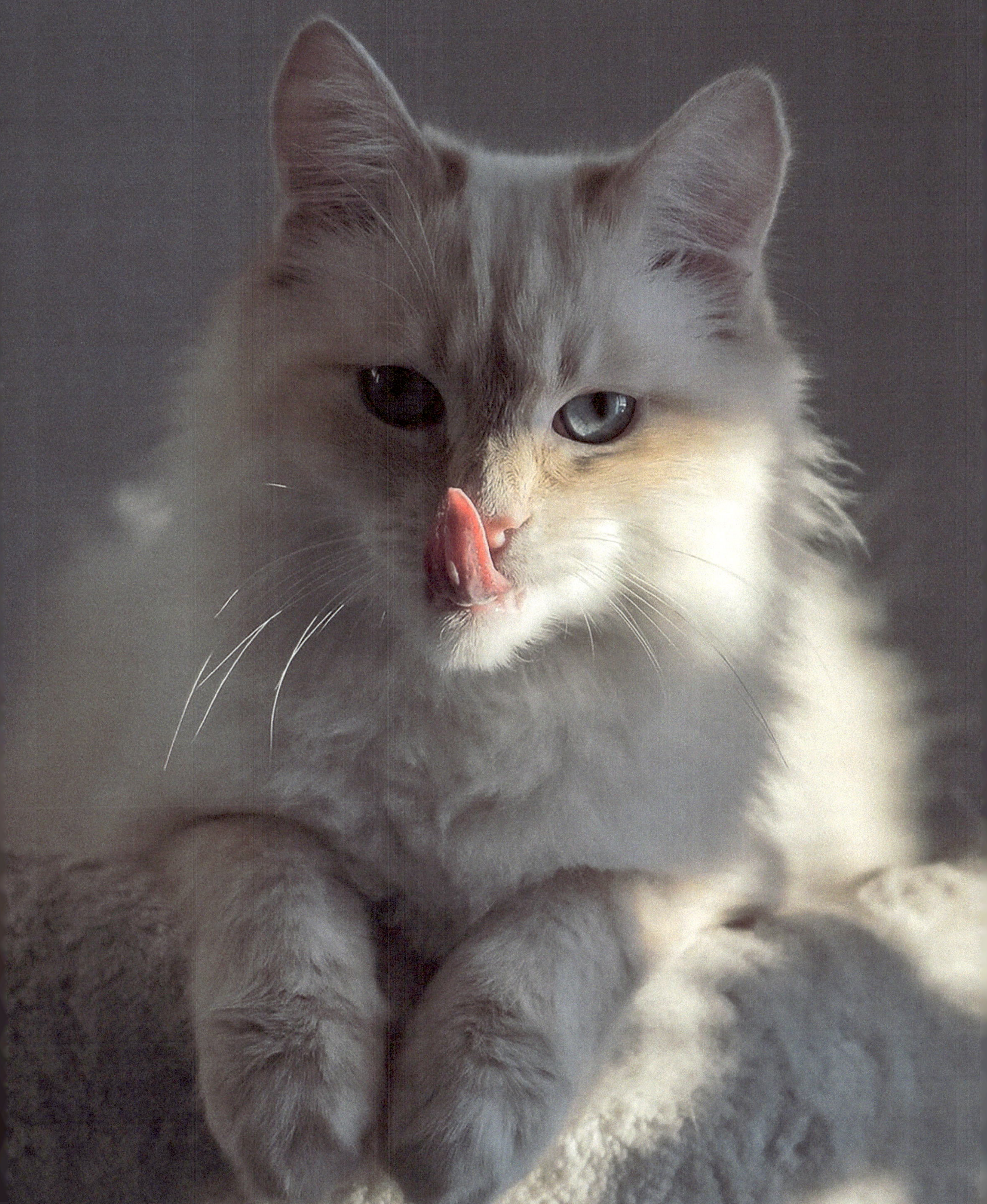

BRITISH LONGHAIR

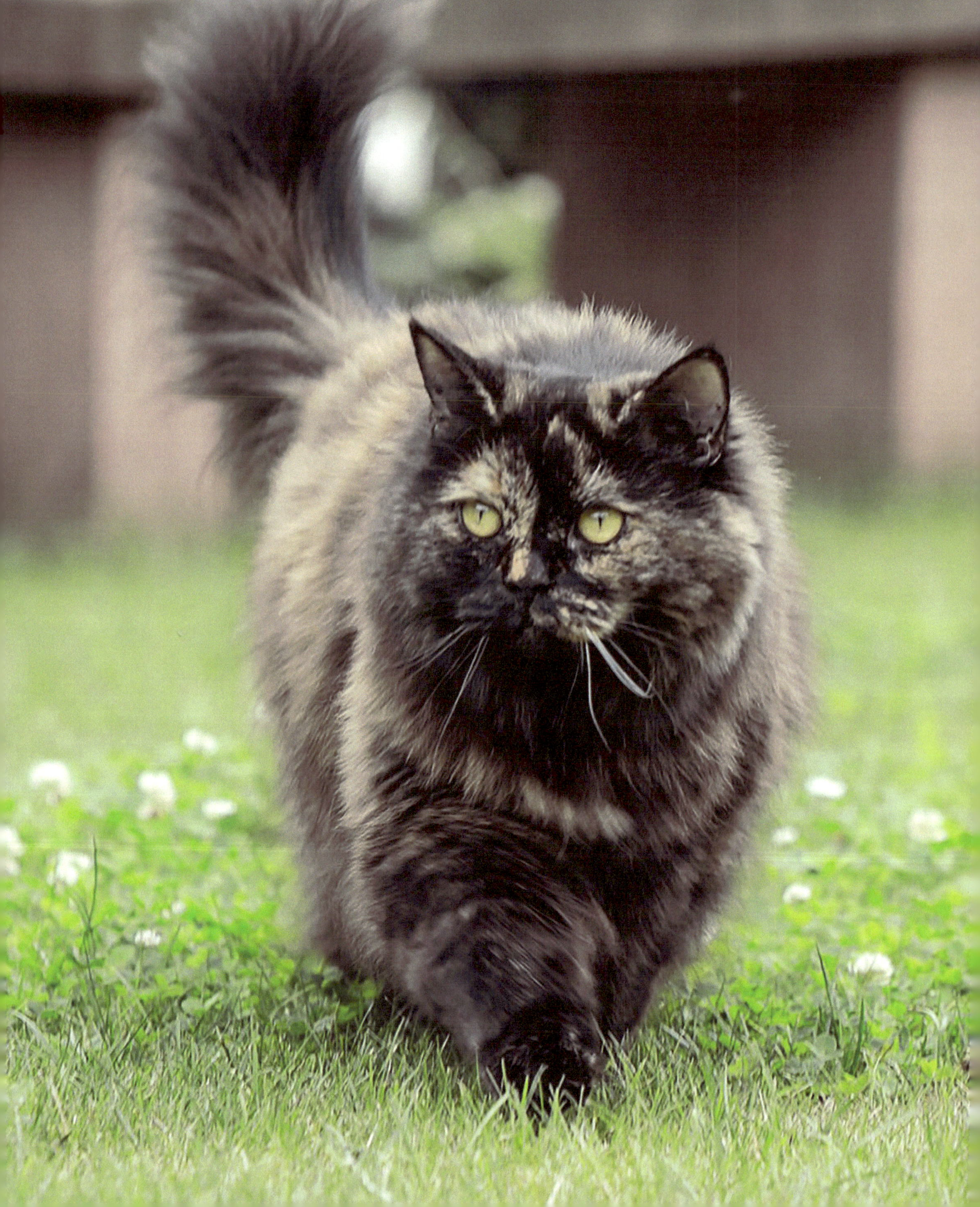

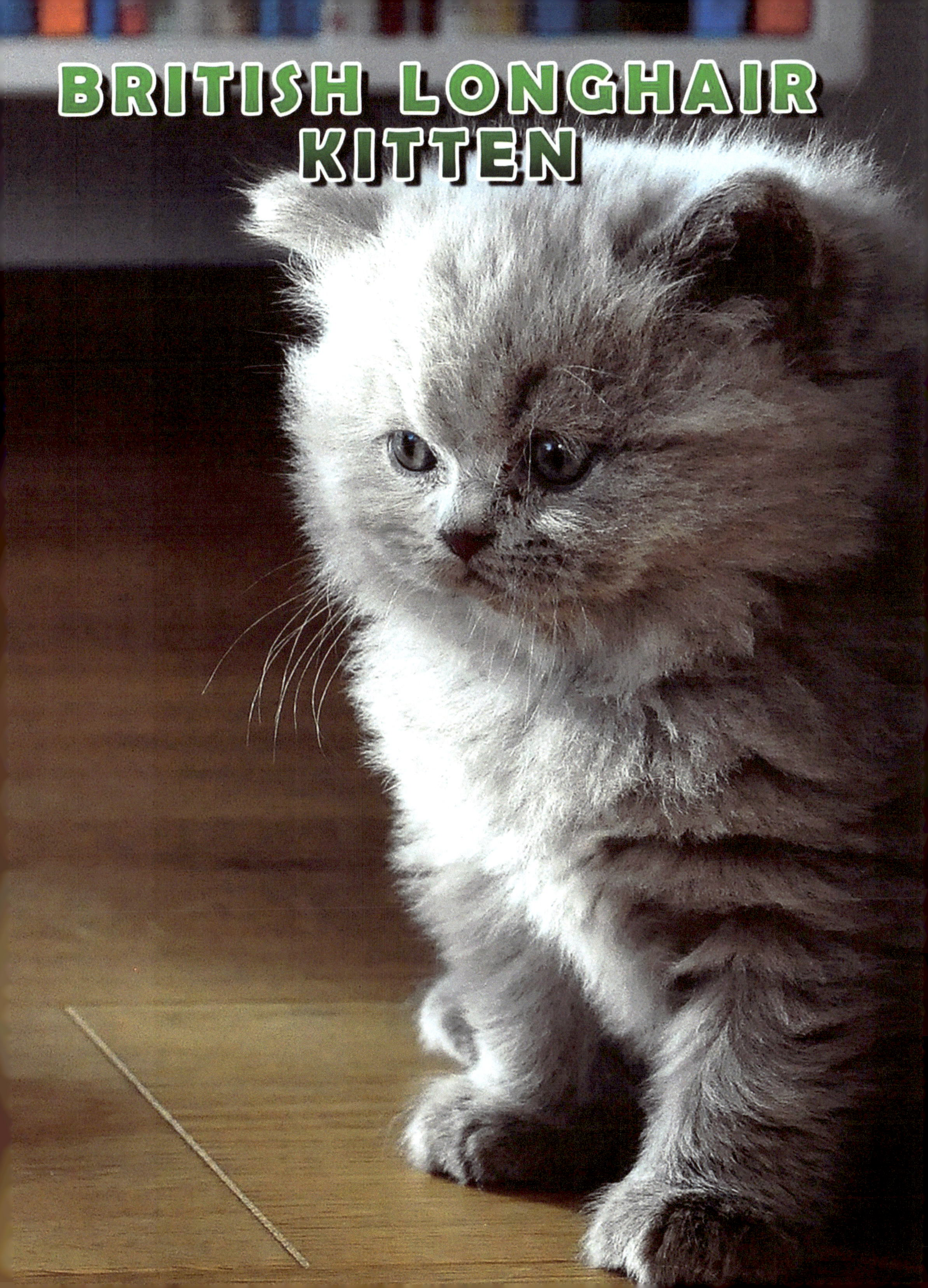
BRITISH LONGHAIR
KITTEN

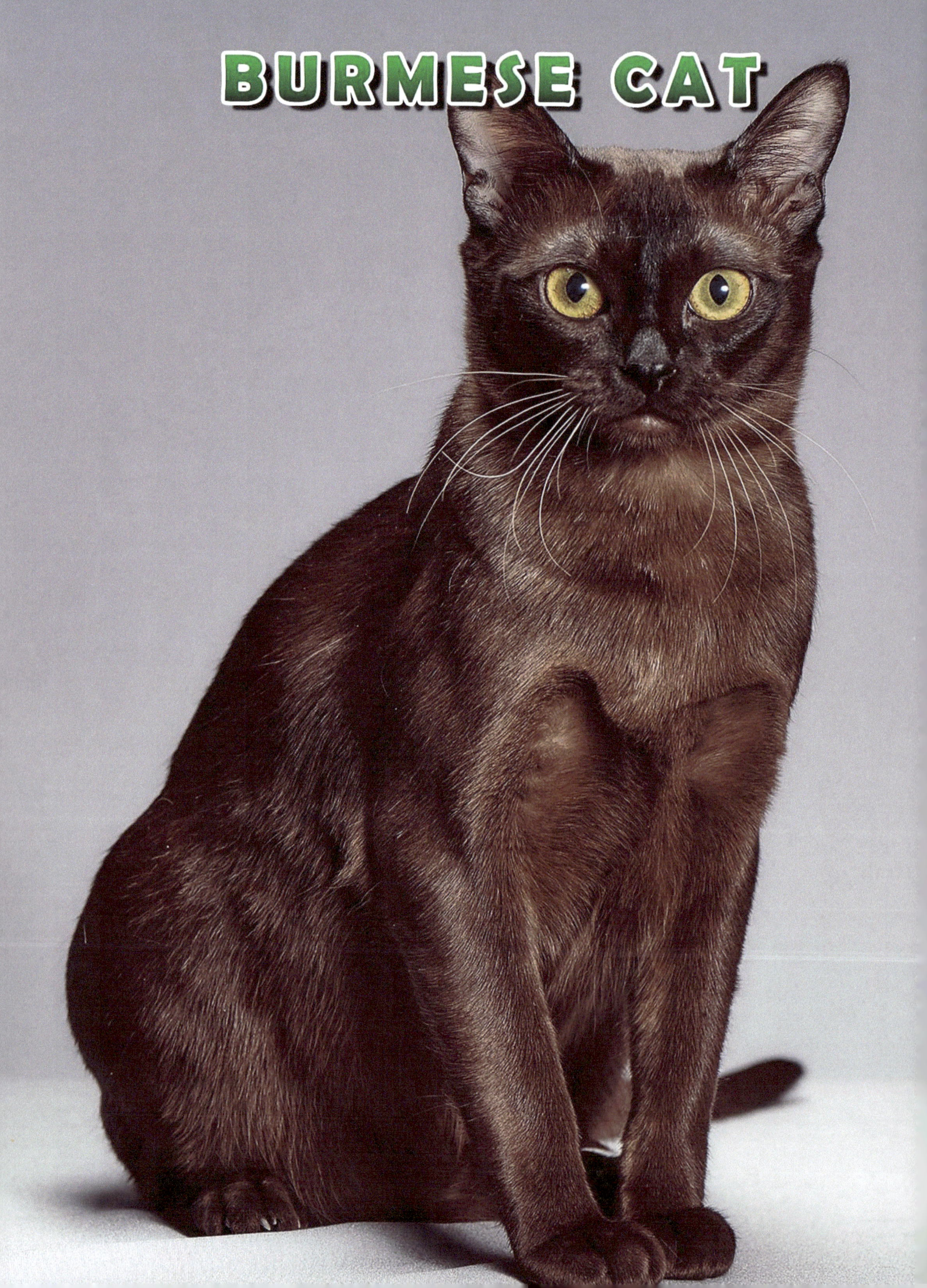

BURMESE CAT

BURMILLA

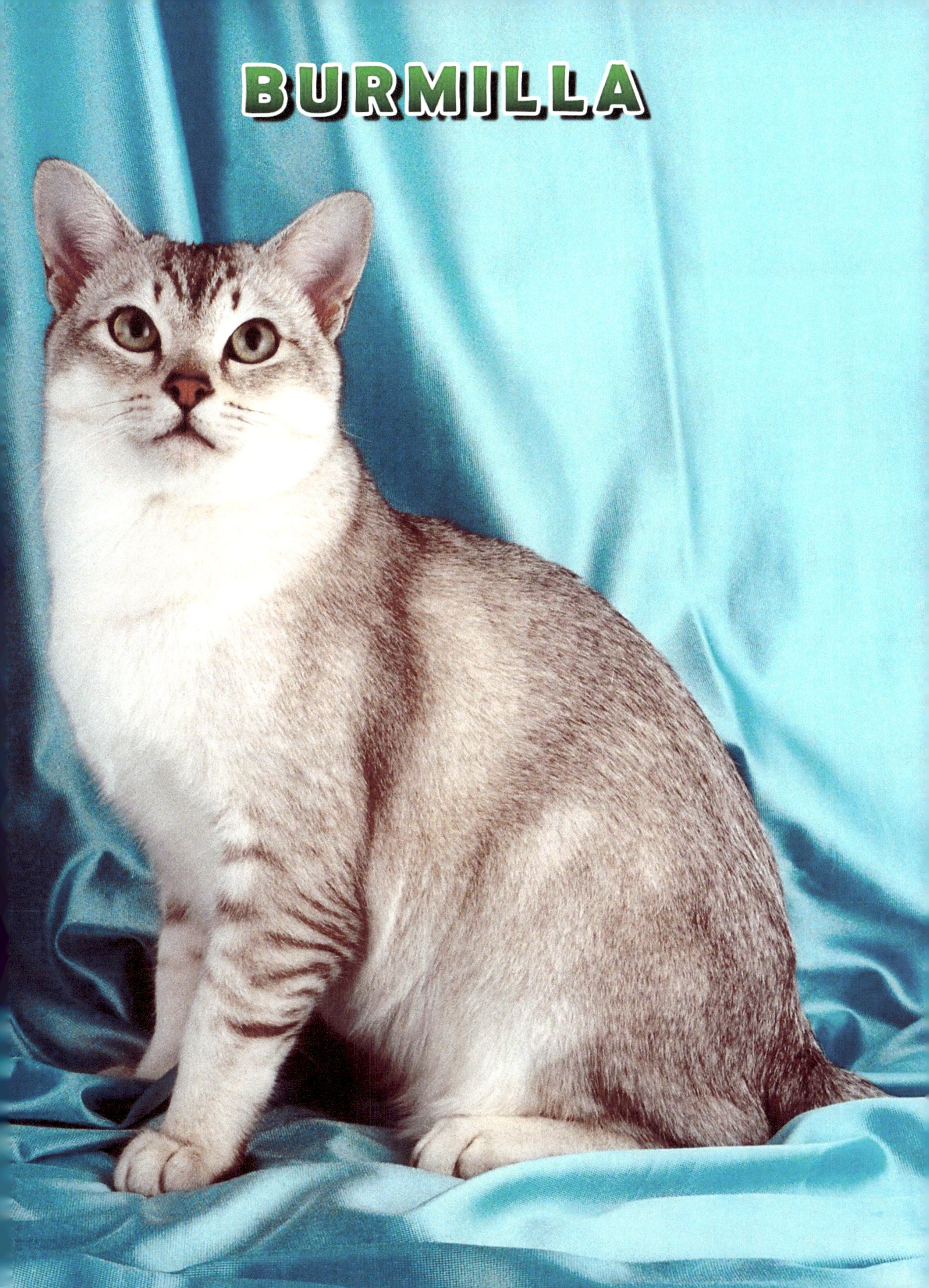

CHARTREUX

CORNISH REX

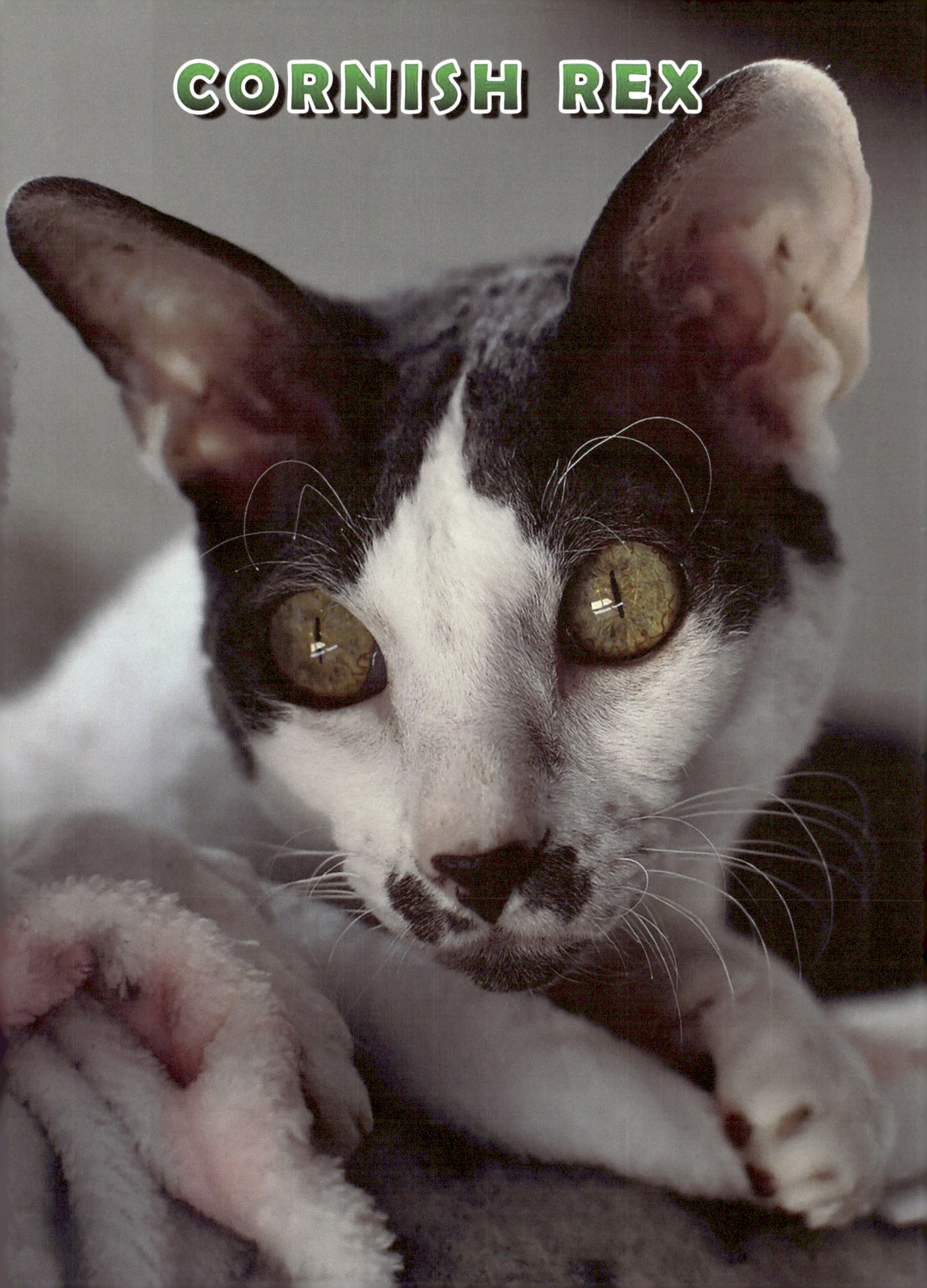

DEVON REX

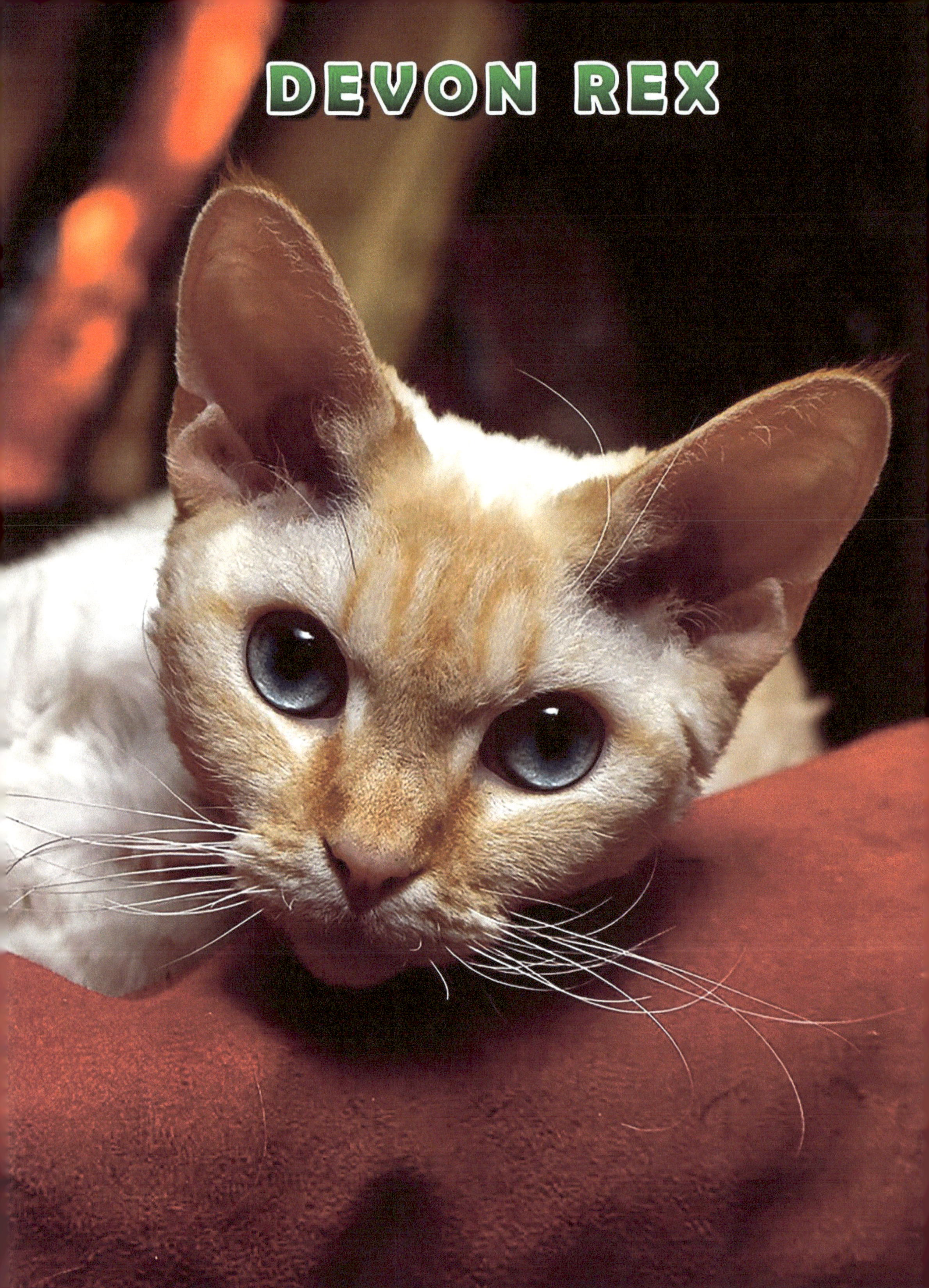

EXOTIC SHORTHAIR KITTEN

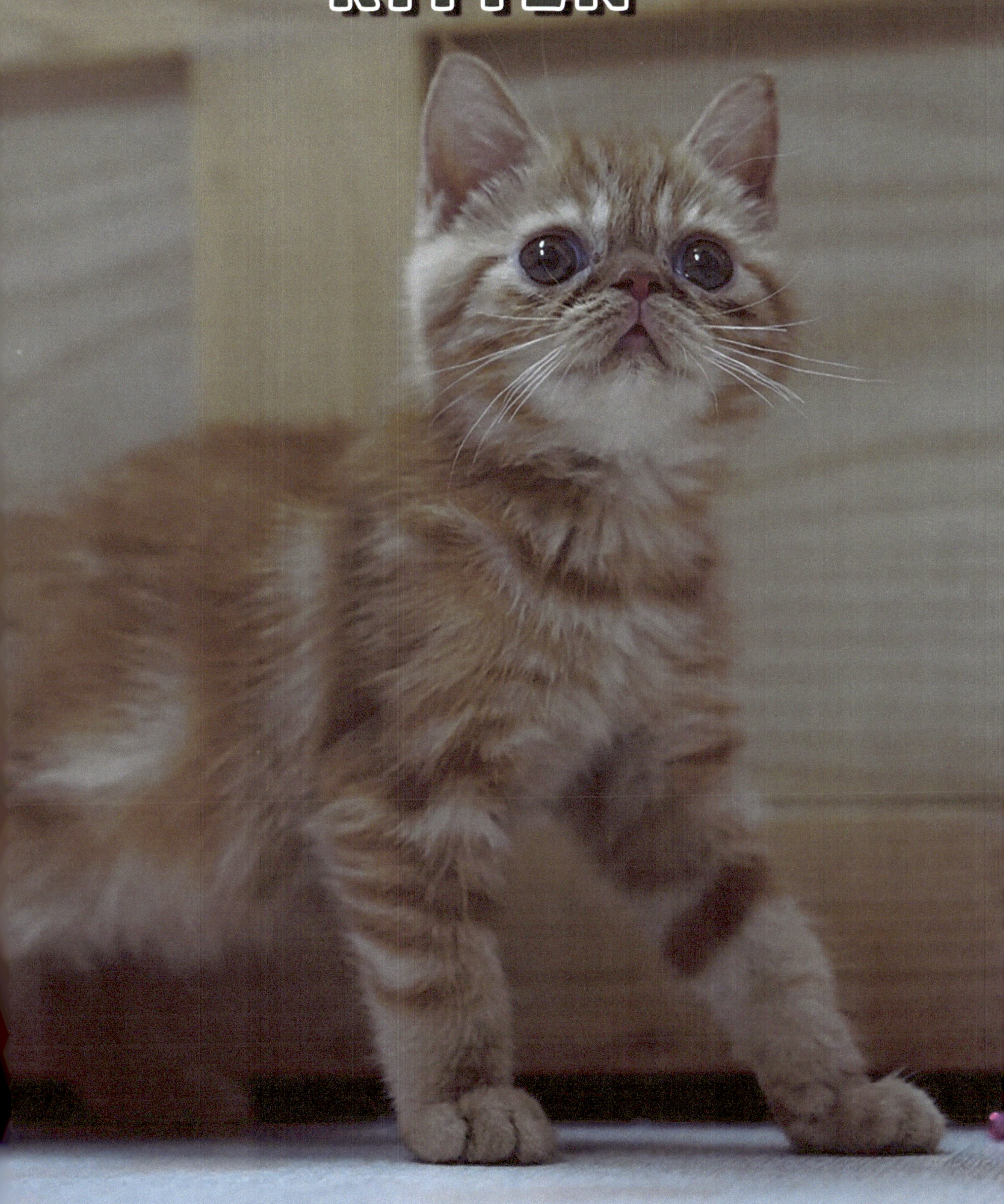

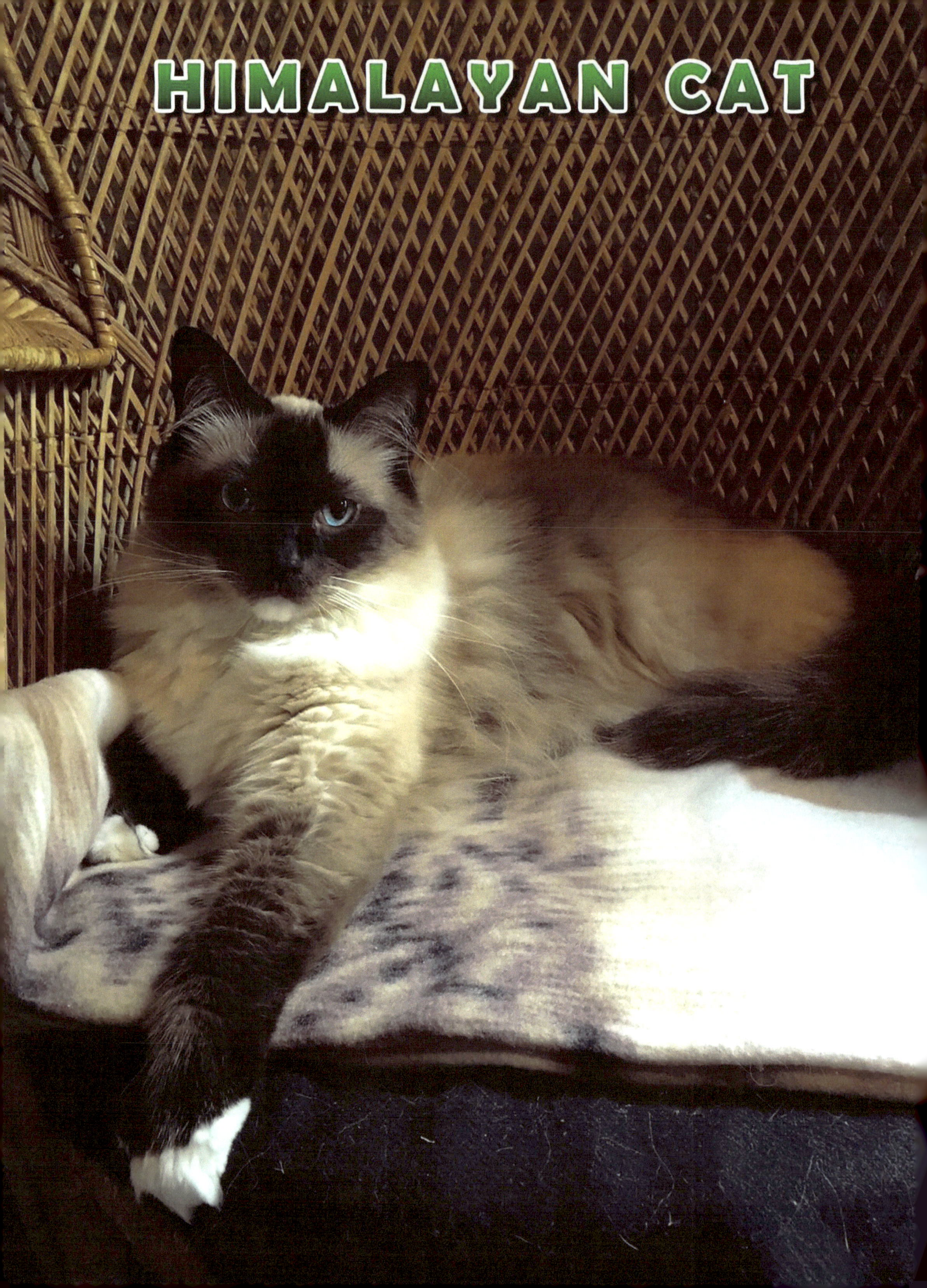

HIMALAYAN CAT

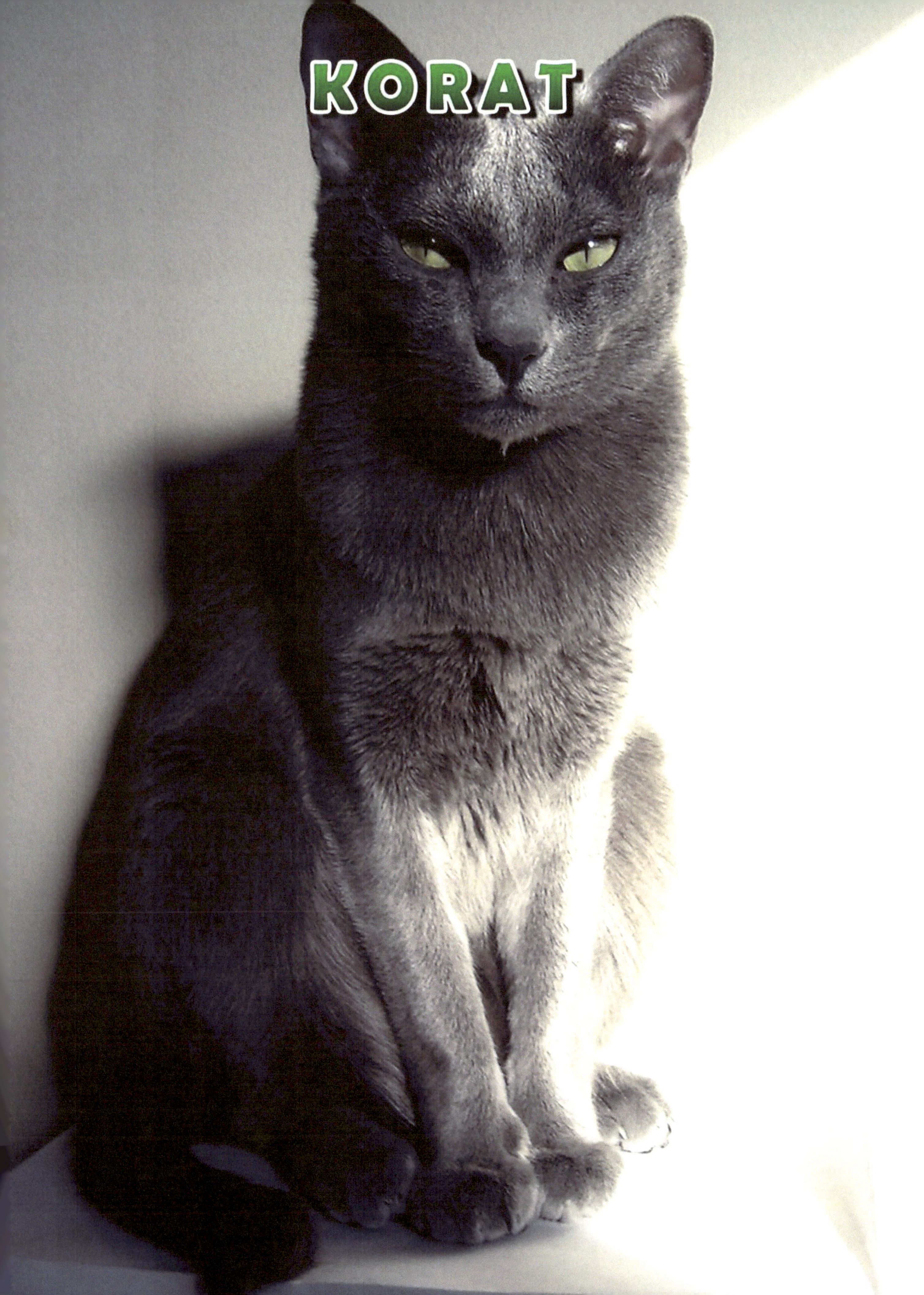

KORAT

KURILIAN BOBTAIL

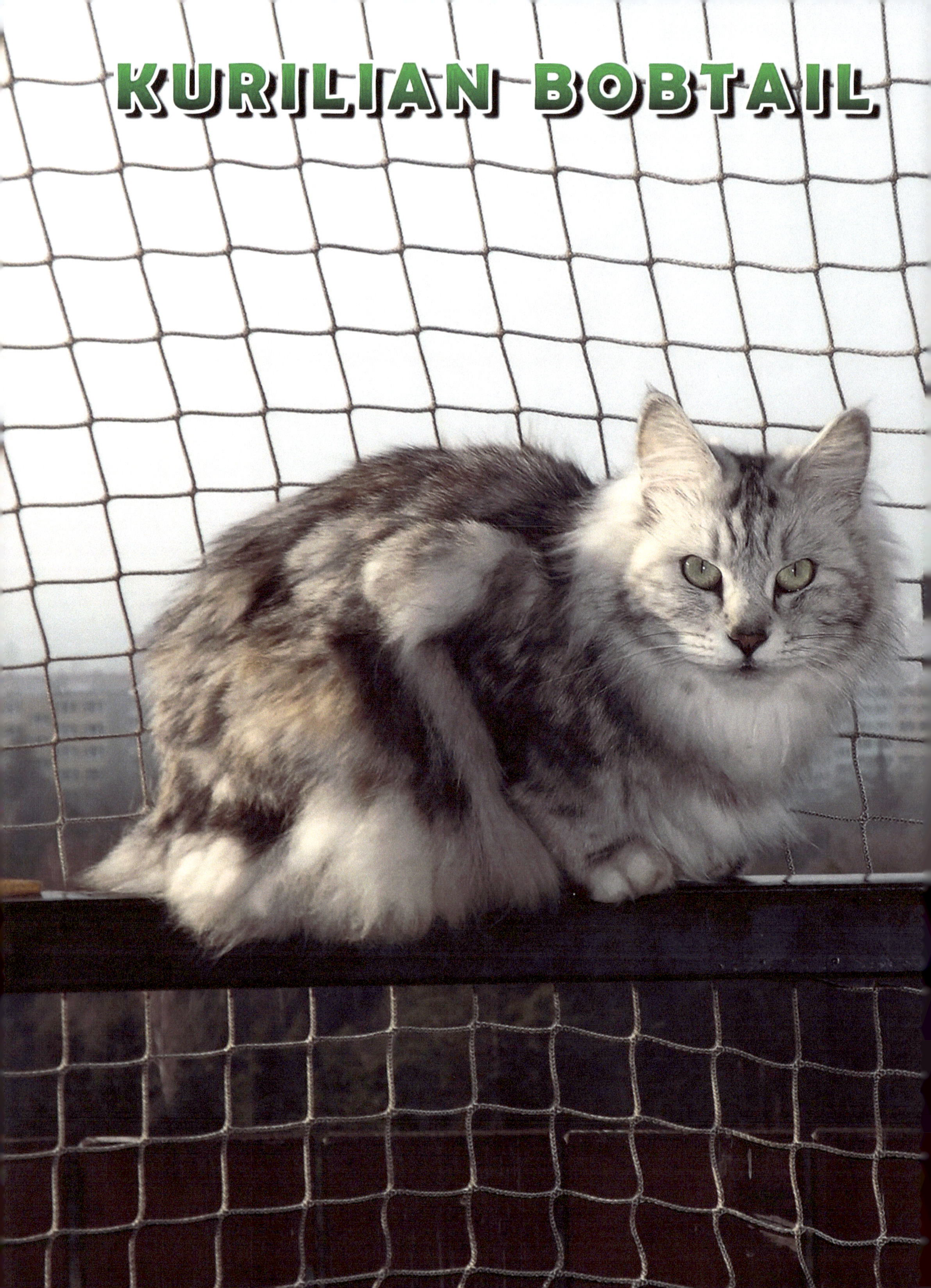

MACKEREL CAT

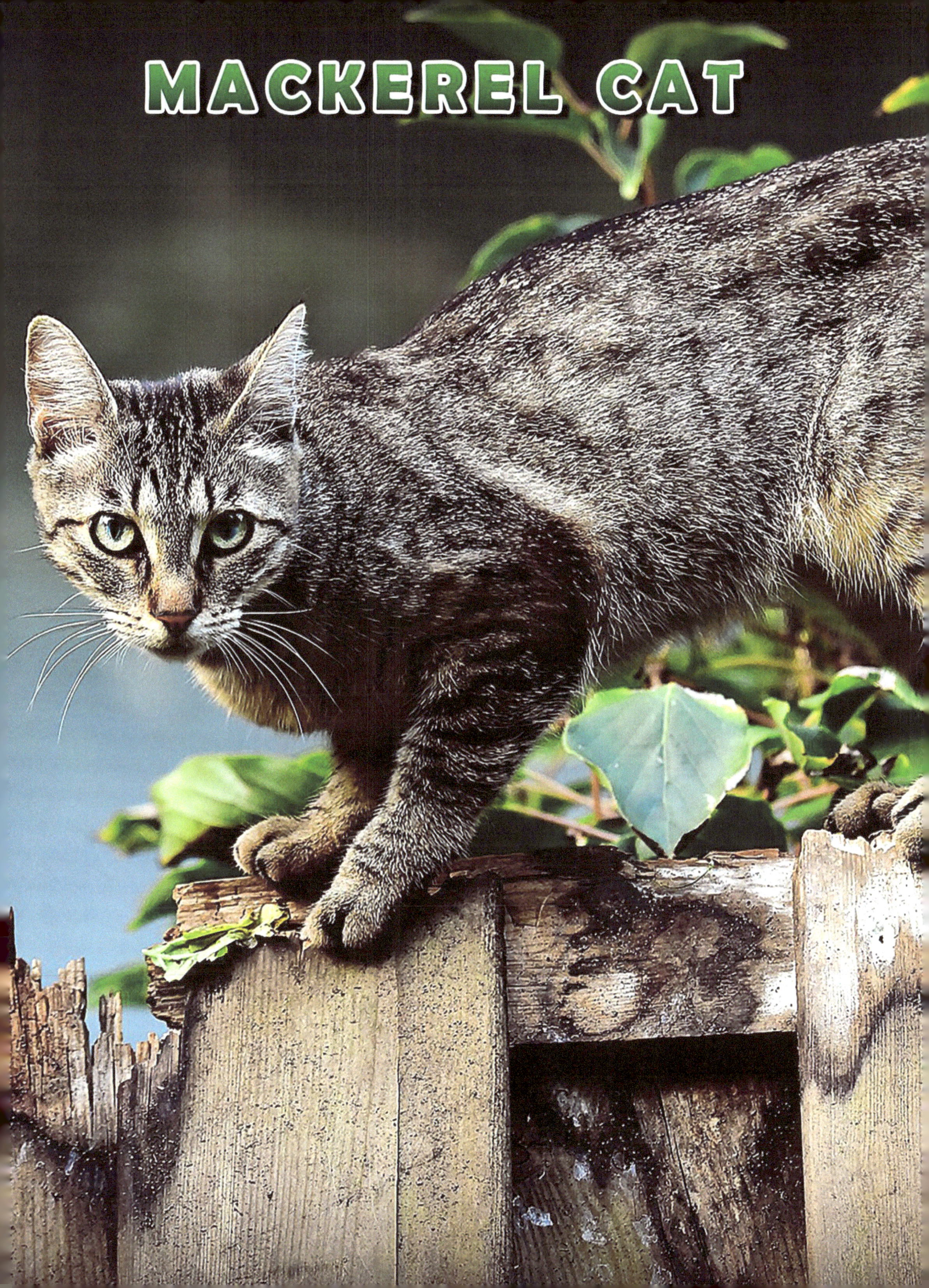

MAINE COON

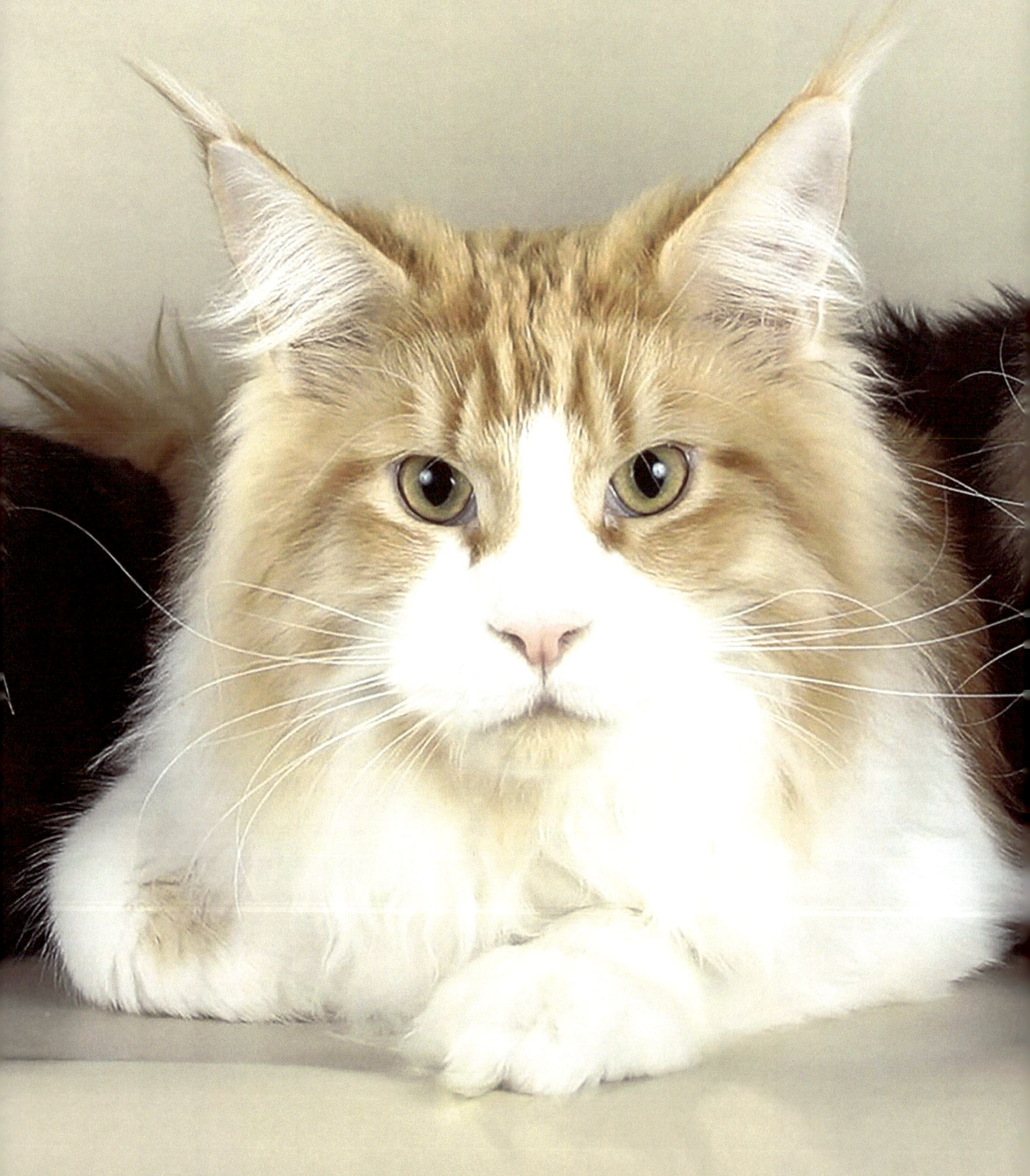

MAINE COON

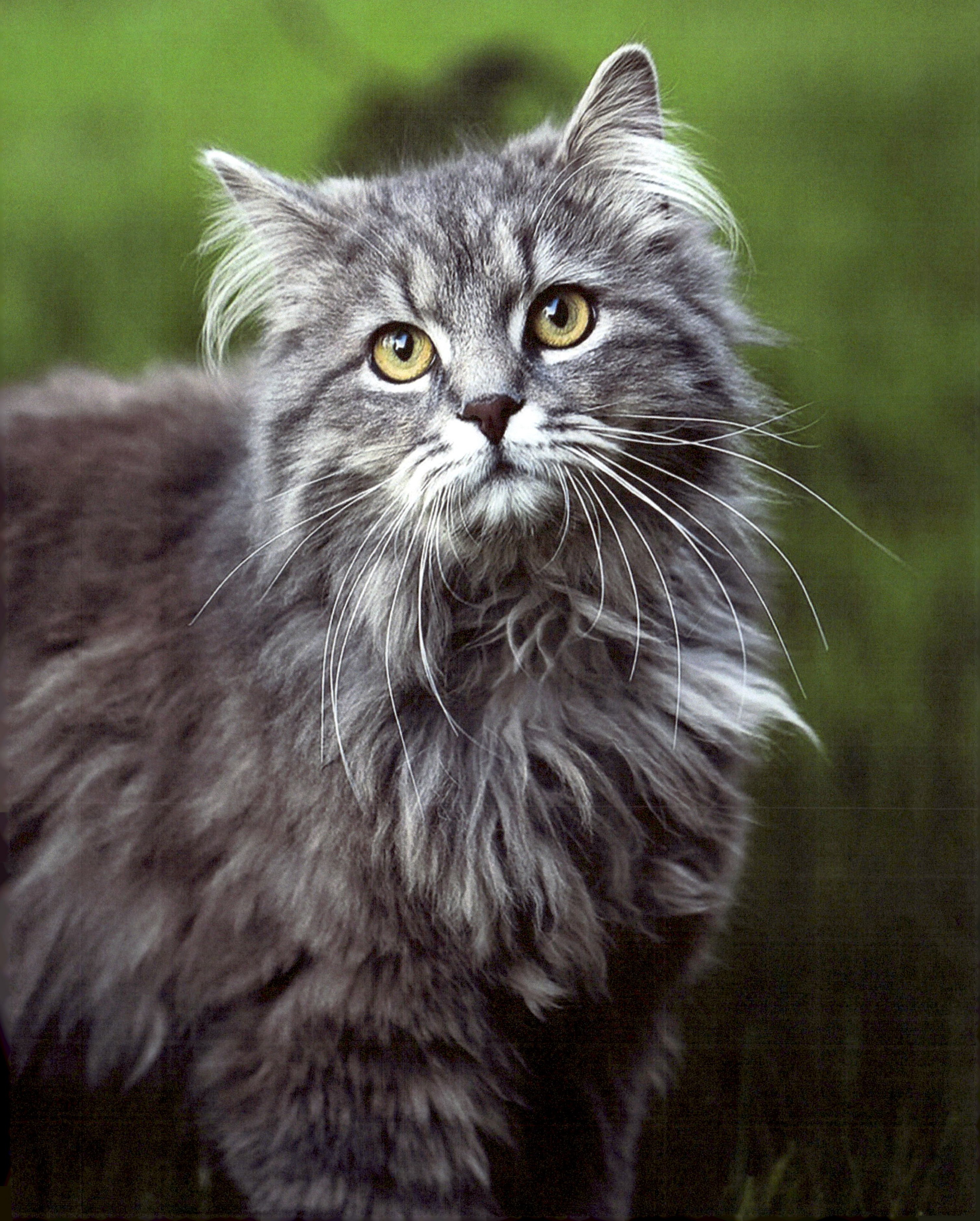

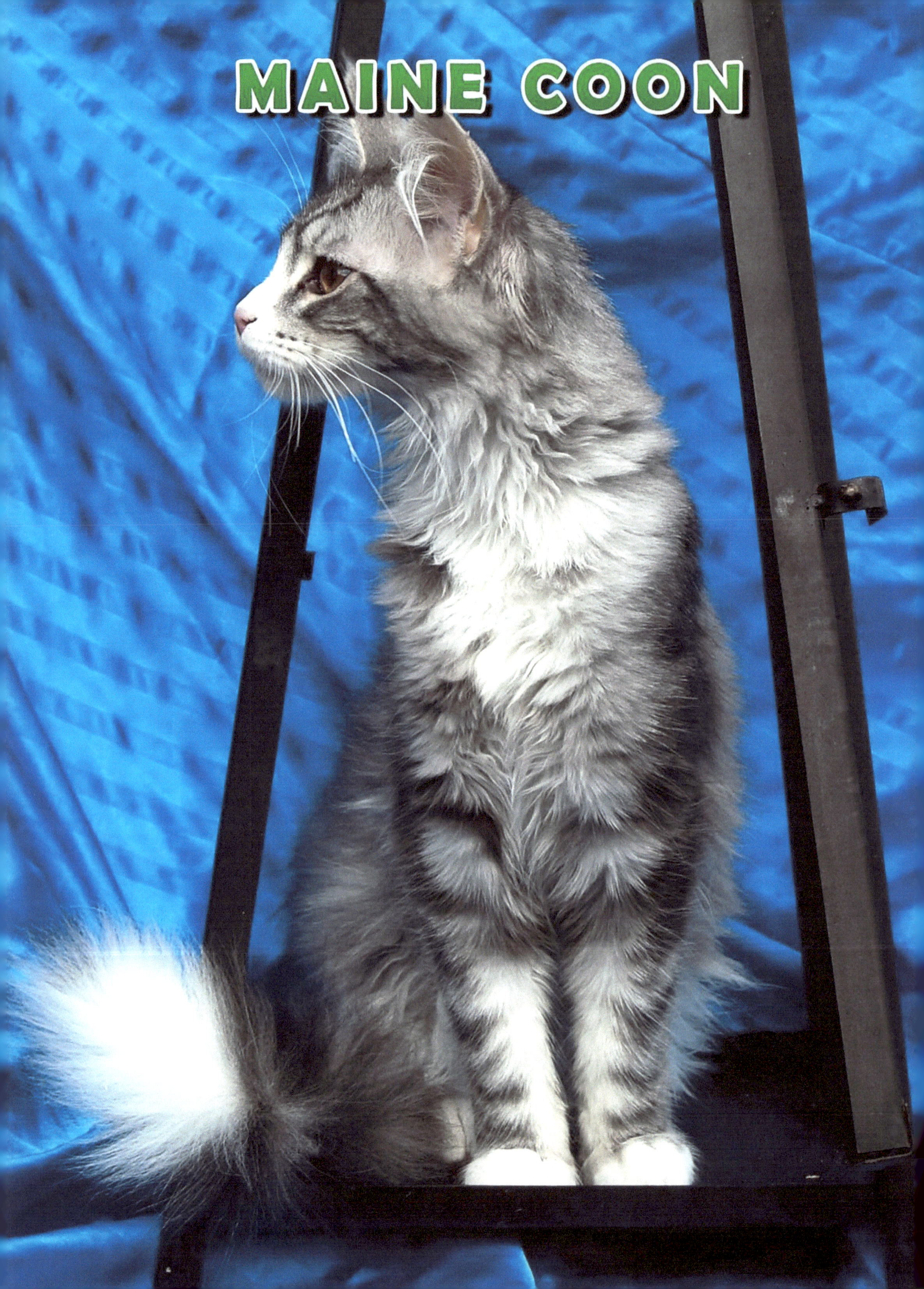

MAINE COON

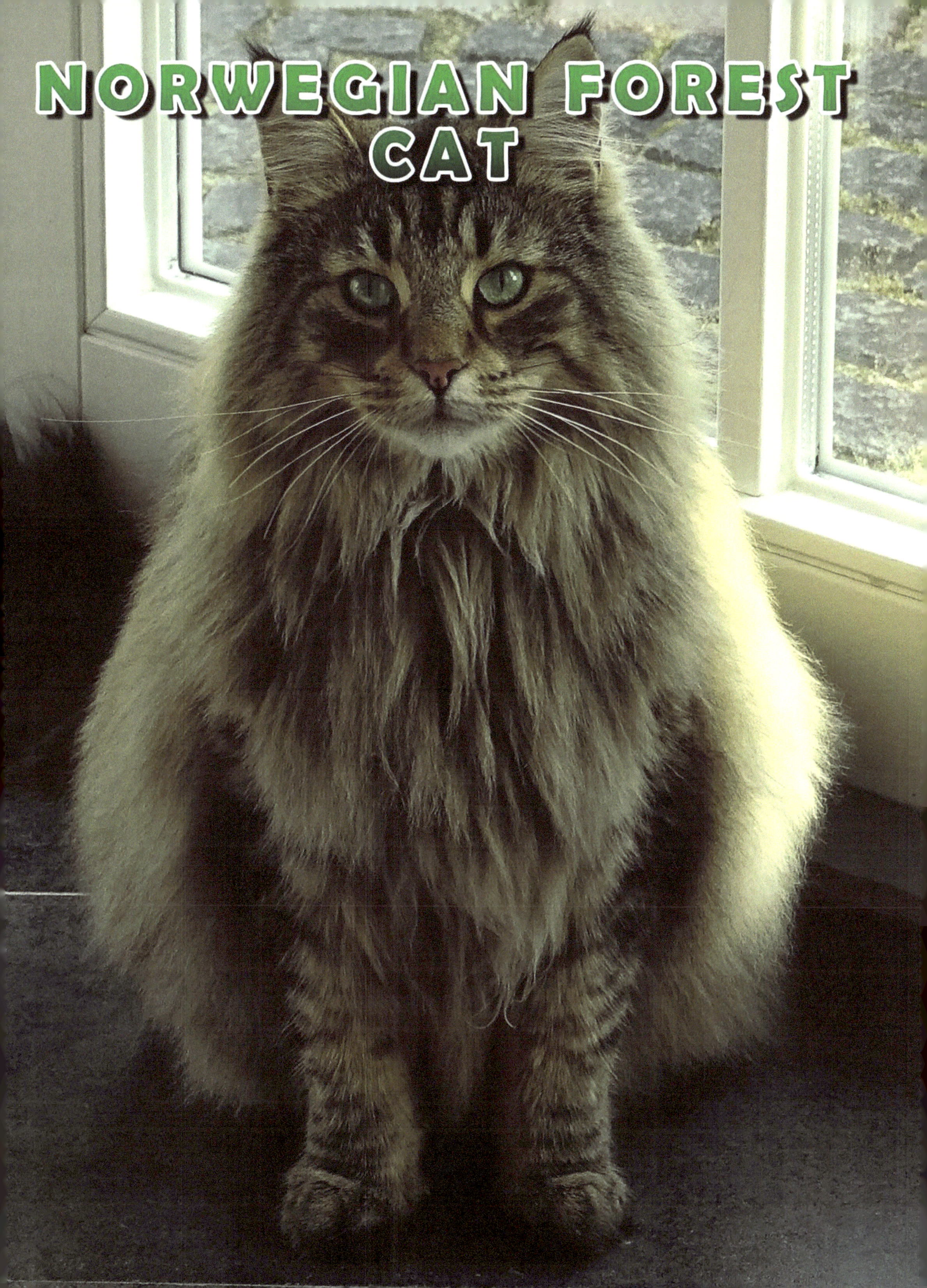
NORWEGIAN FOREST
CAT

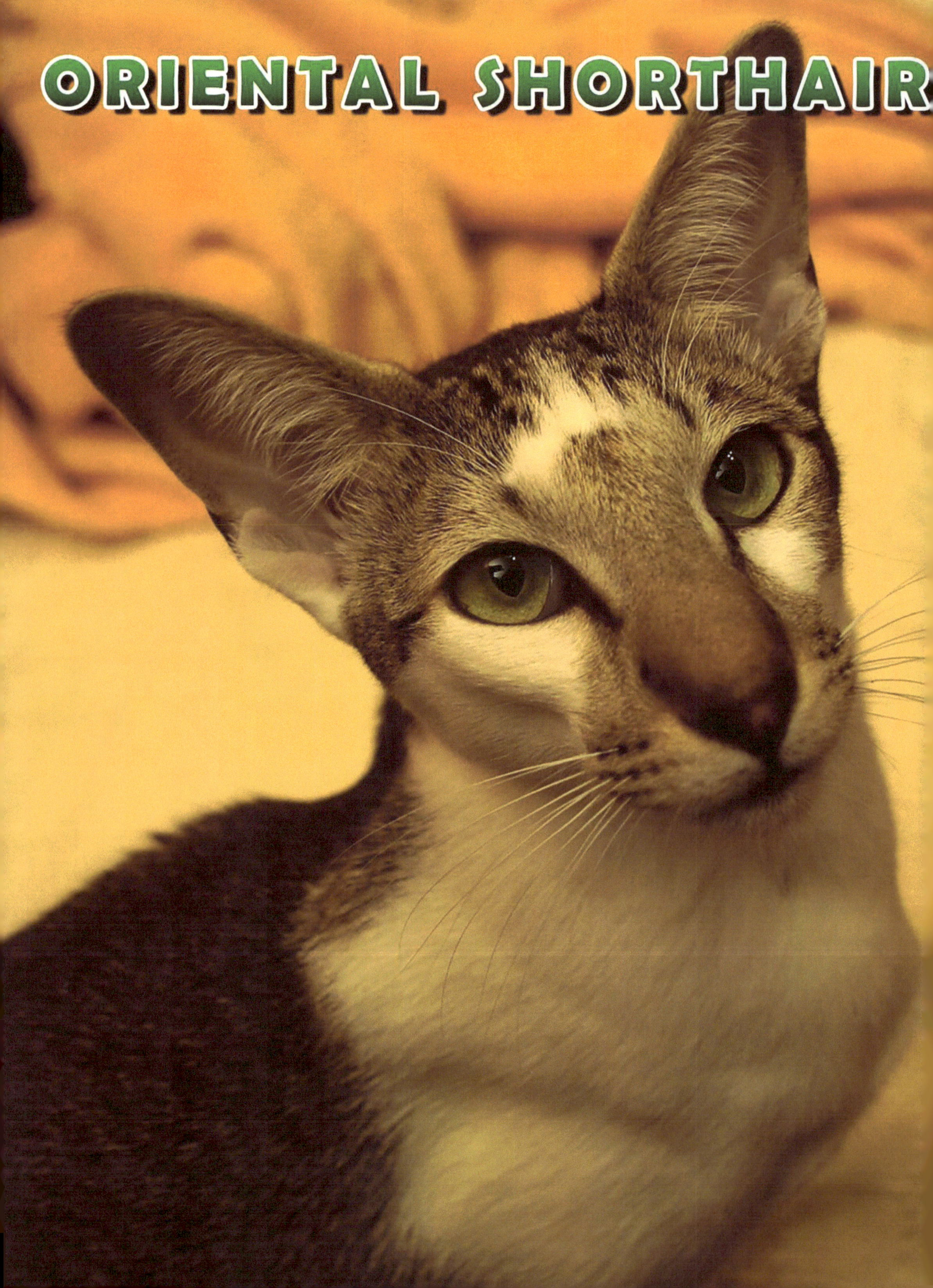
ORIENTAL SHORTHAIR

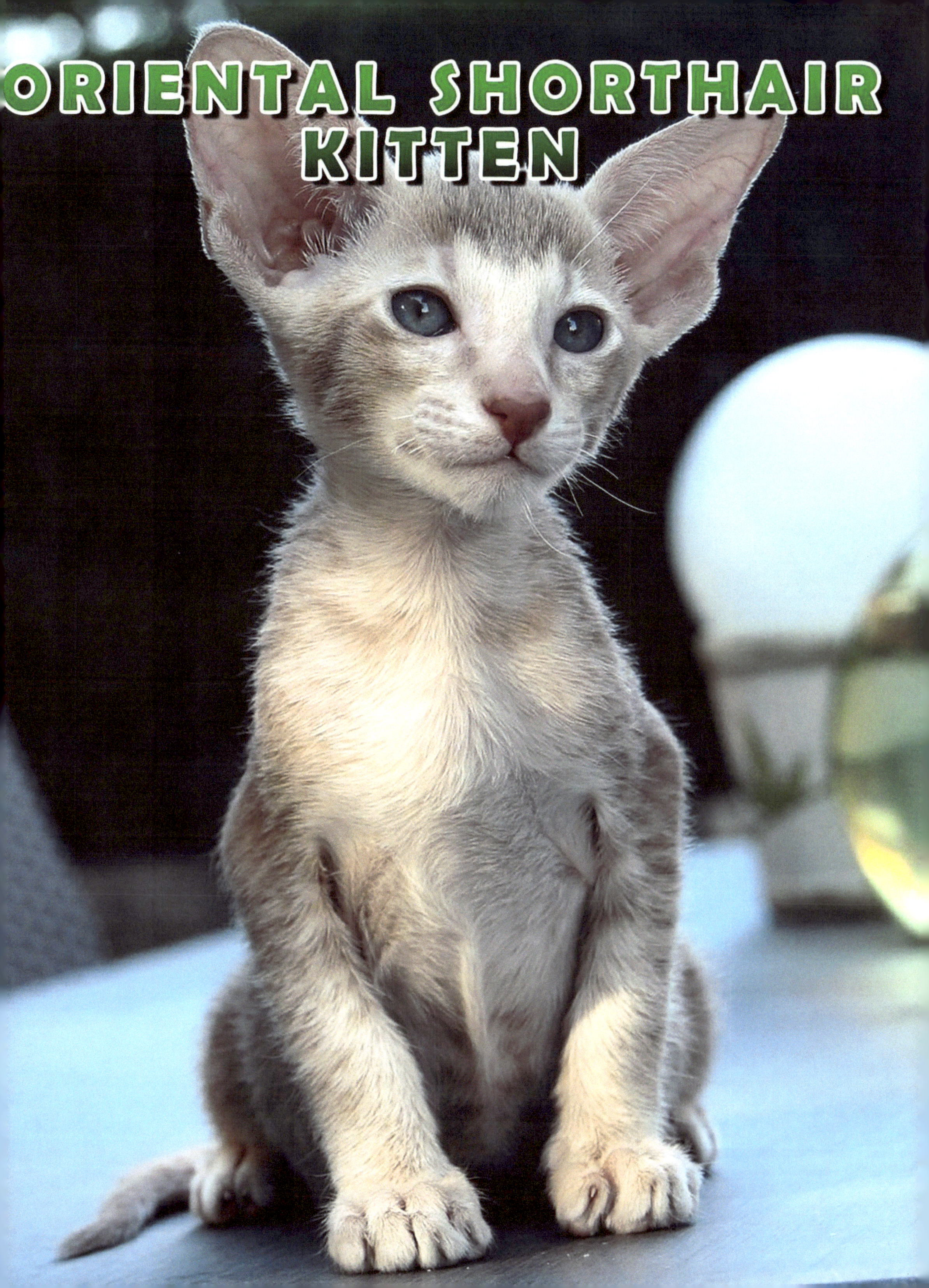
ORIENTAL SHORTHAIR
KITTEN

PERSIAN CAT

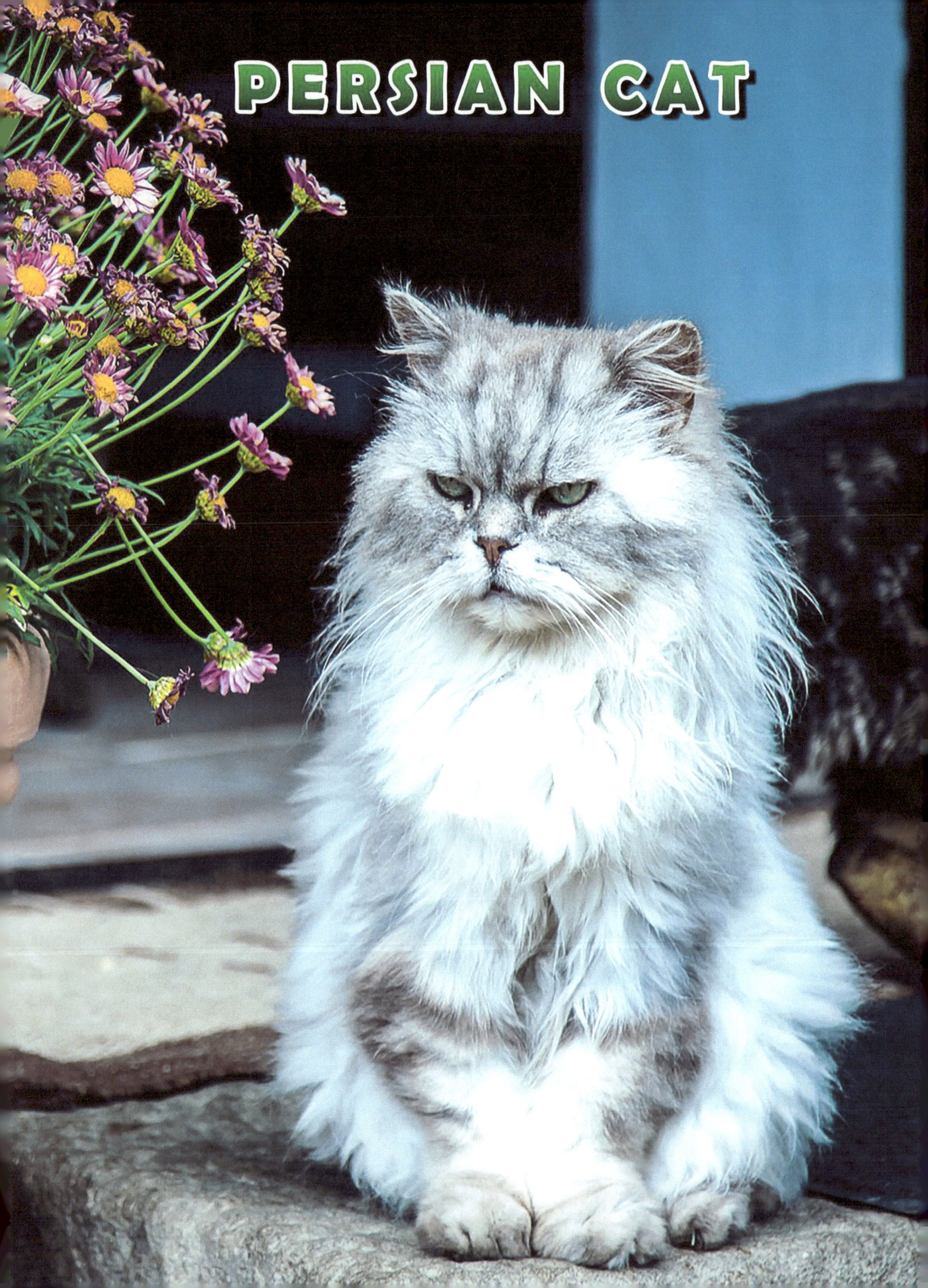

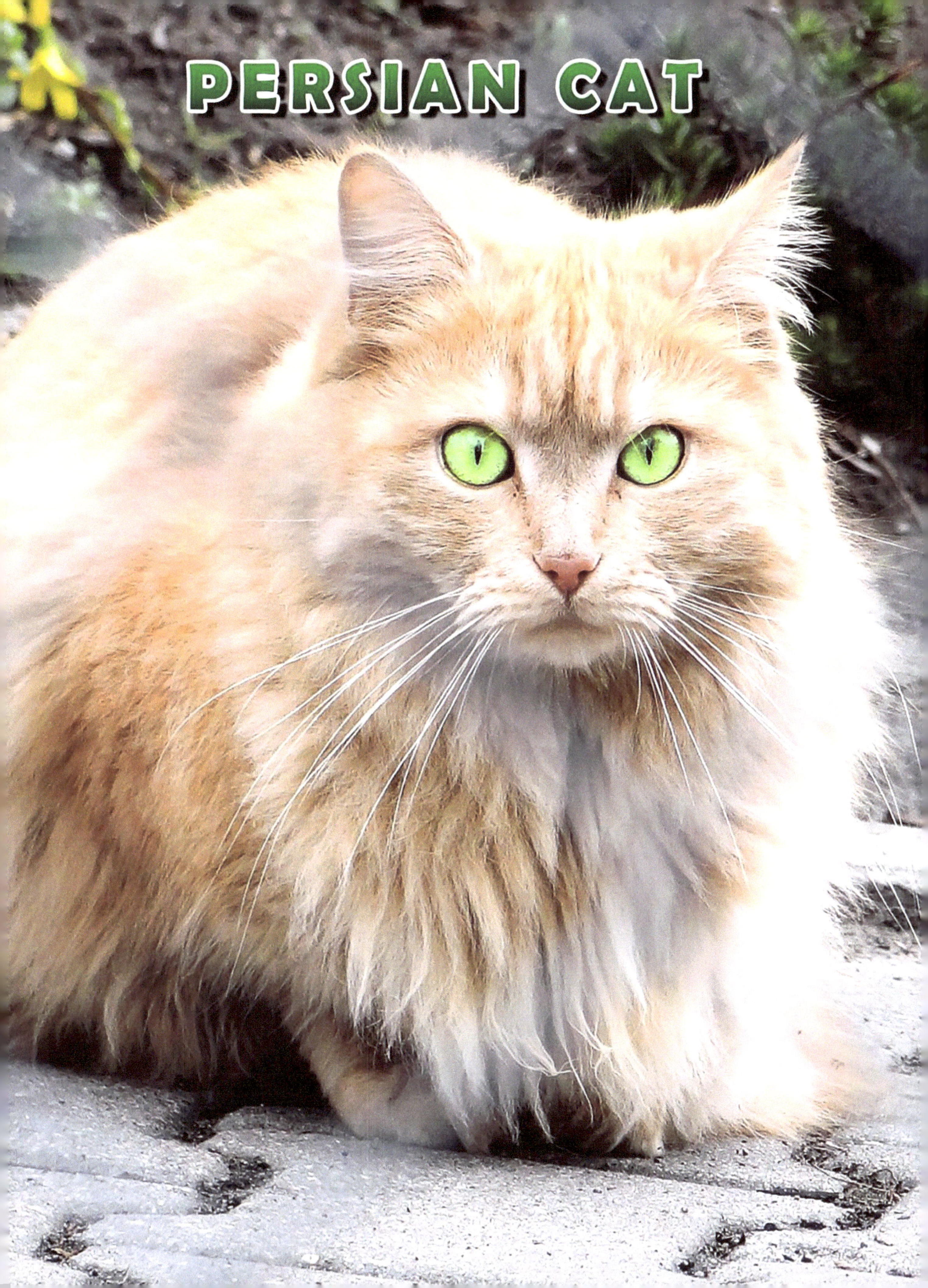
PERSIAN CAT

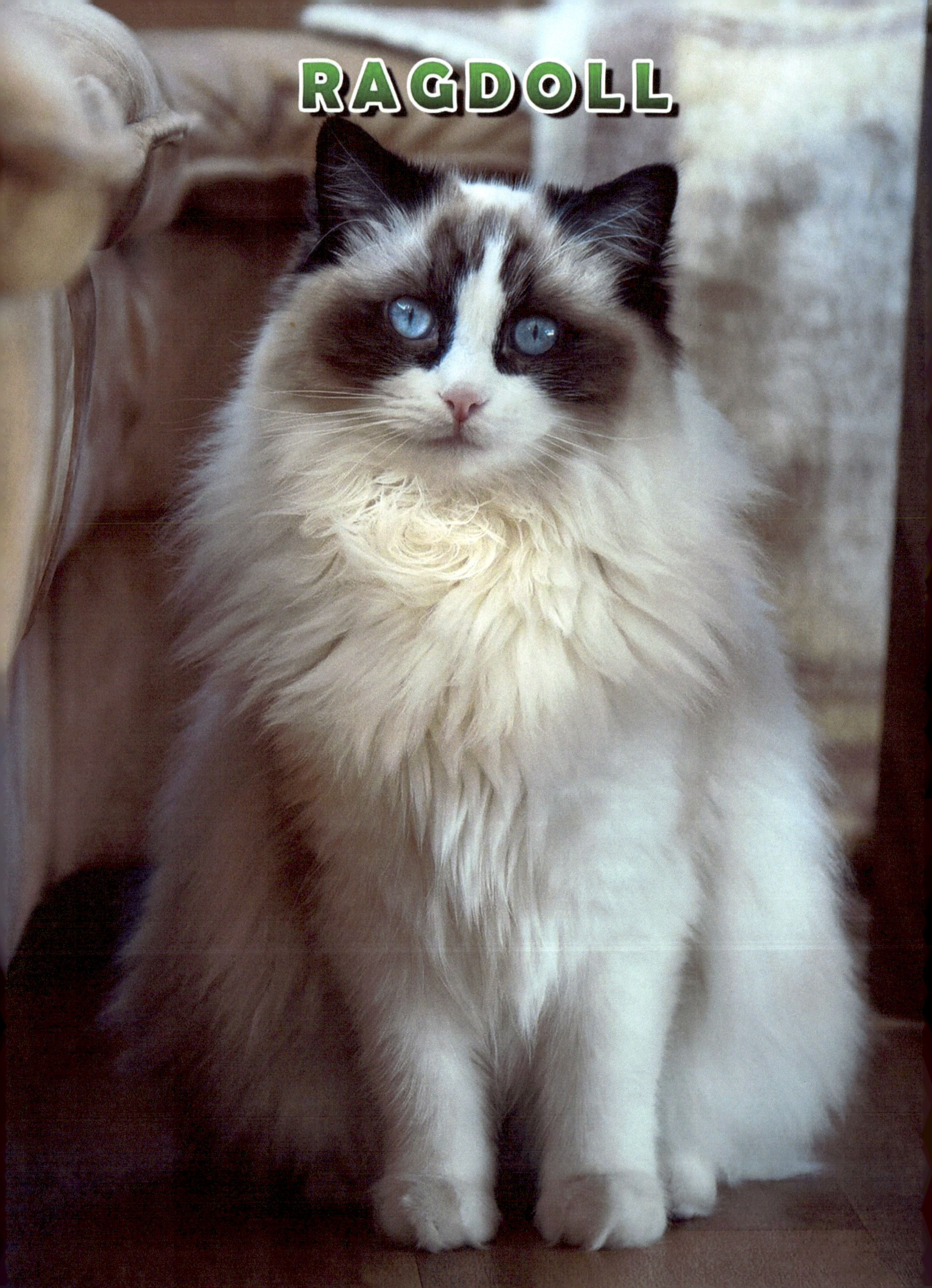
RAGDOLL

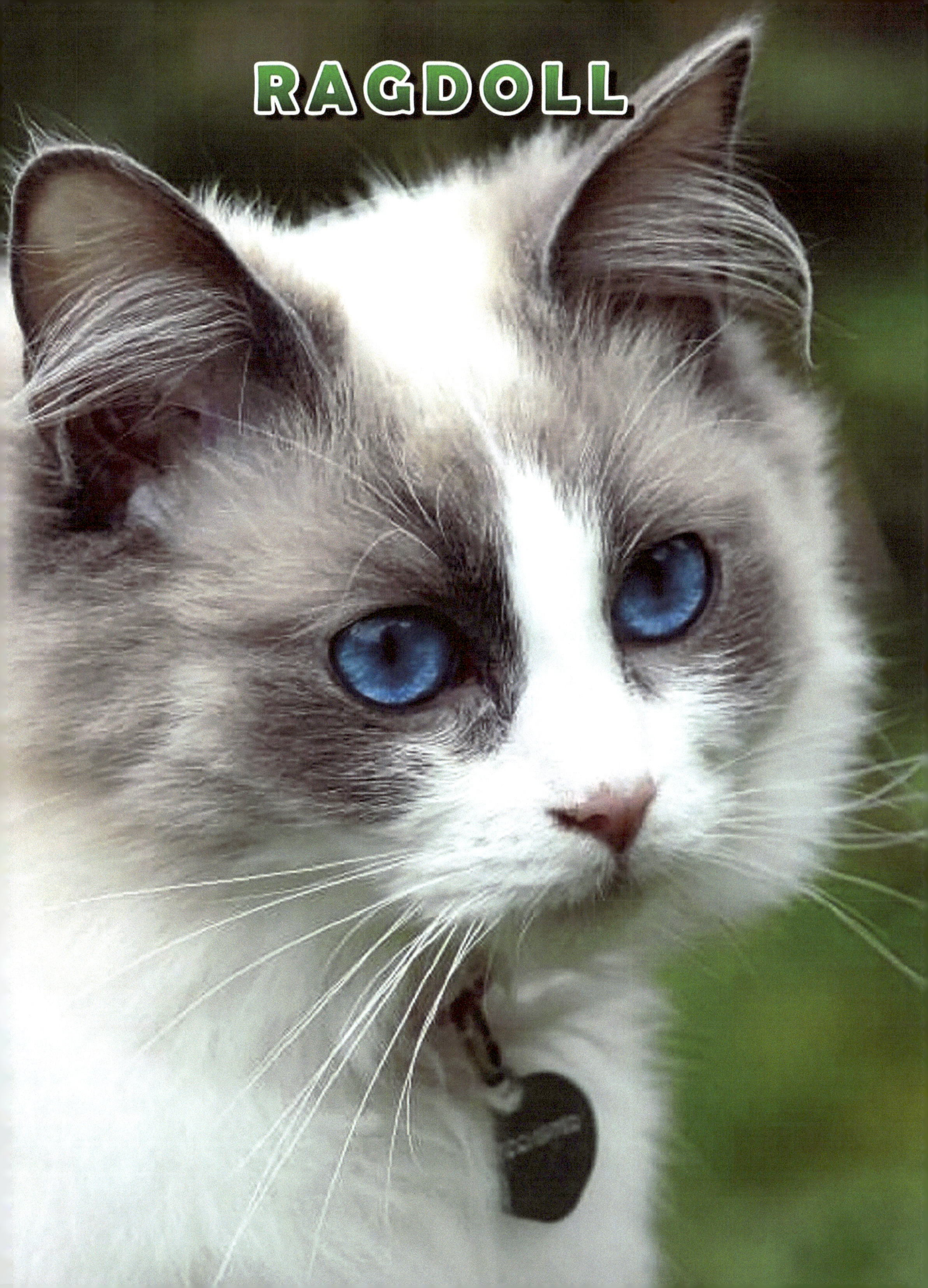
RAGDOLL

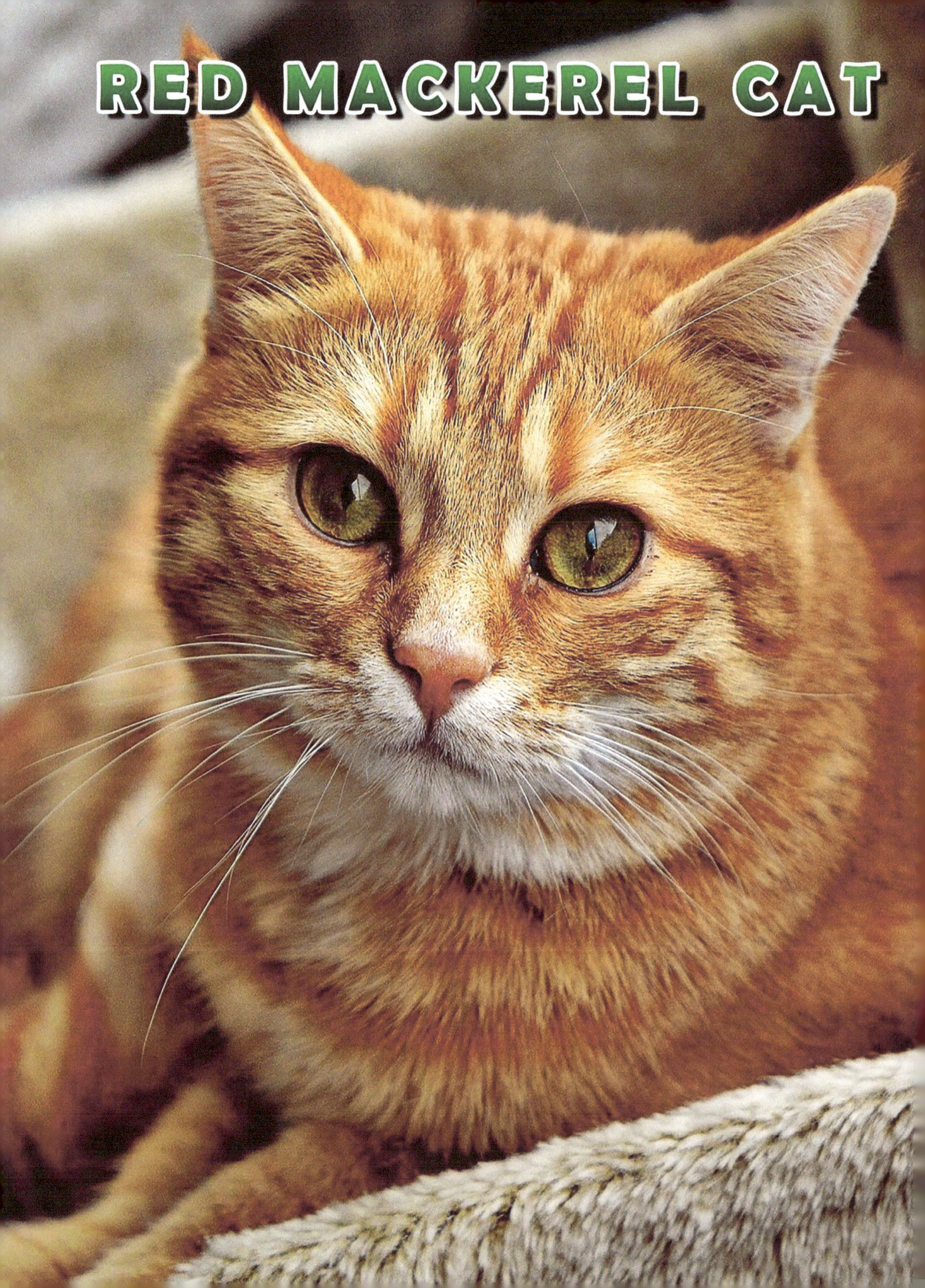
RED MACKEREL CAT

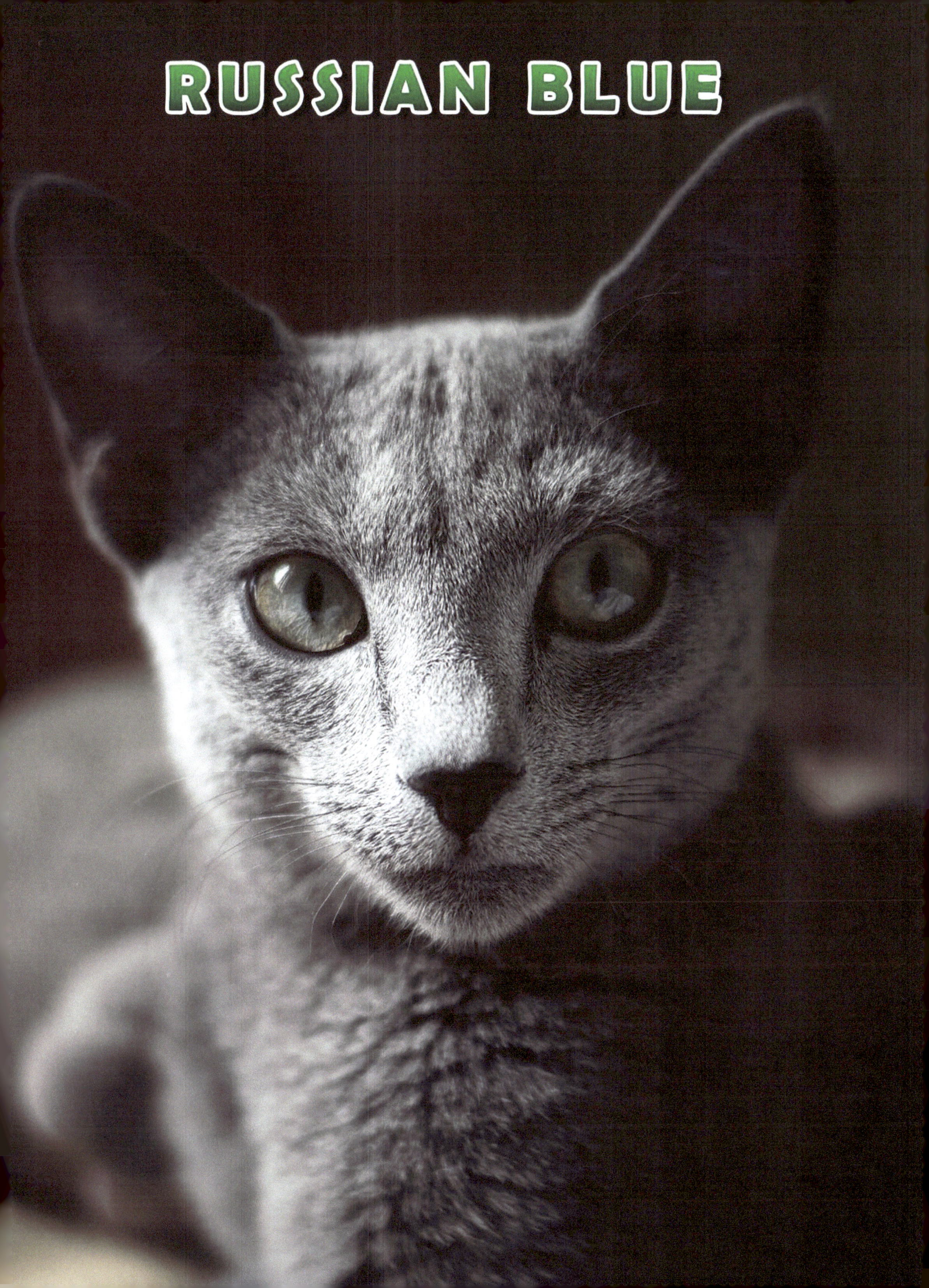

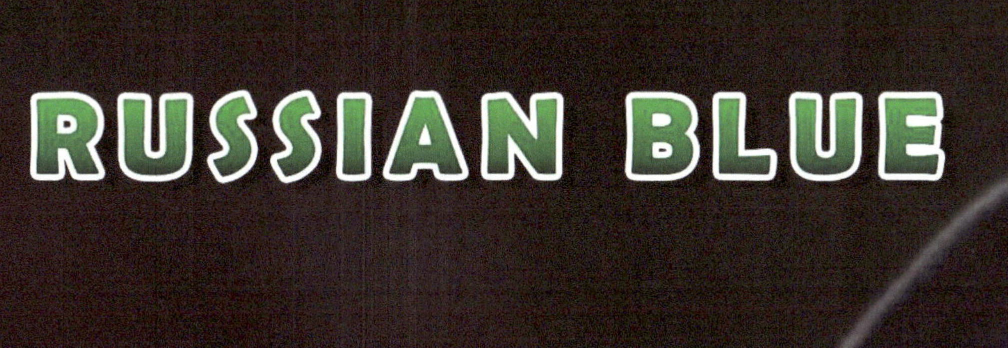
RUSSIAN BLUE

RUSSIAN BLUE

SAVANNAH CAT

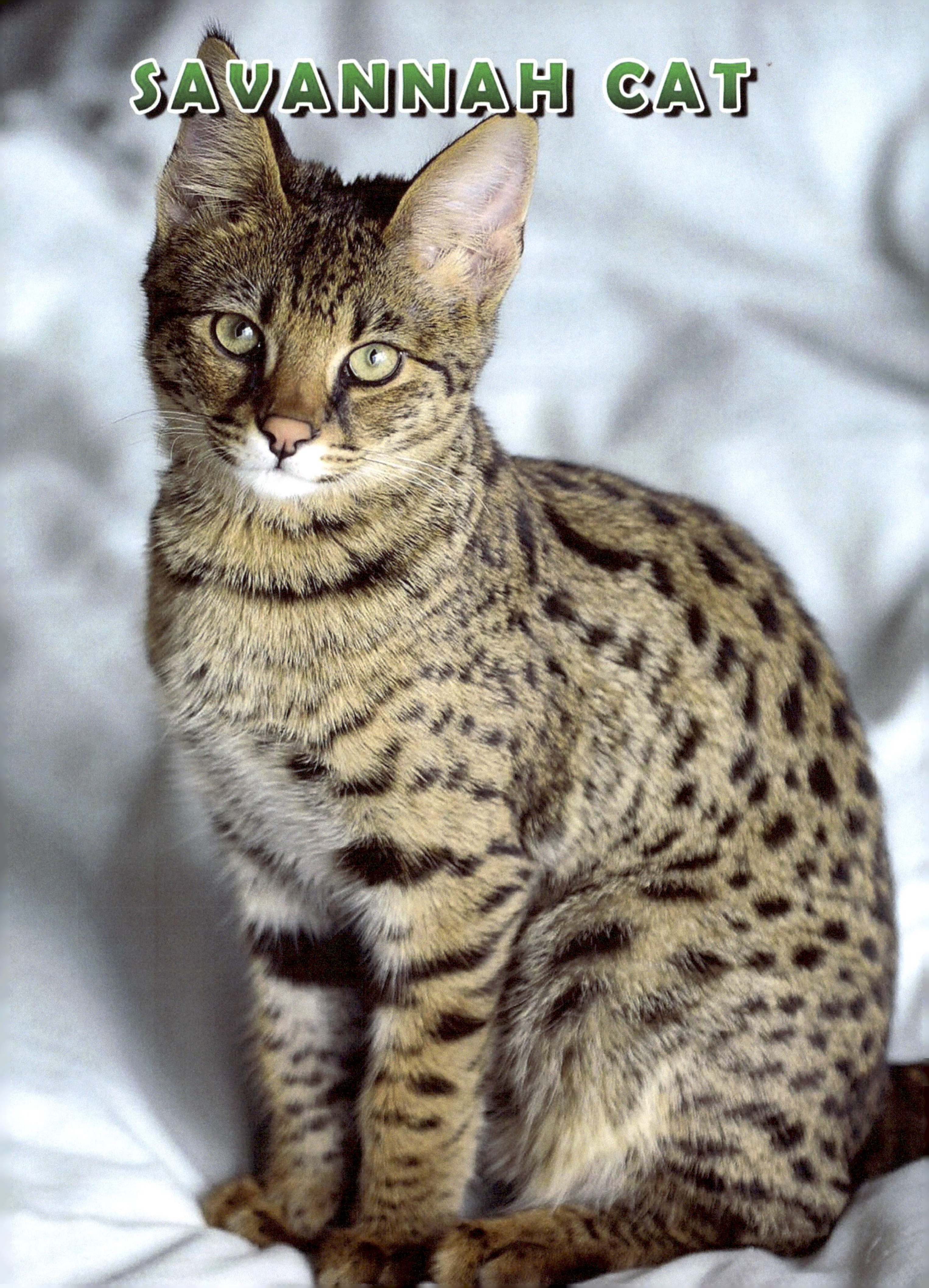

SCOTTISH FOLD

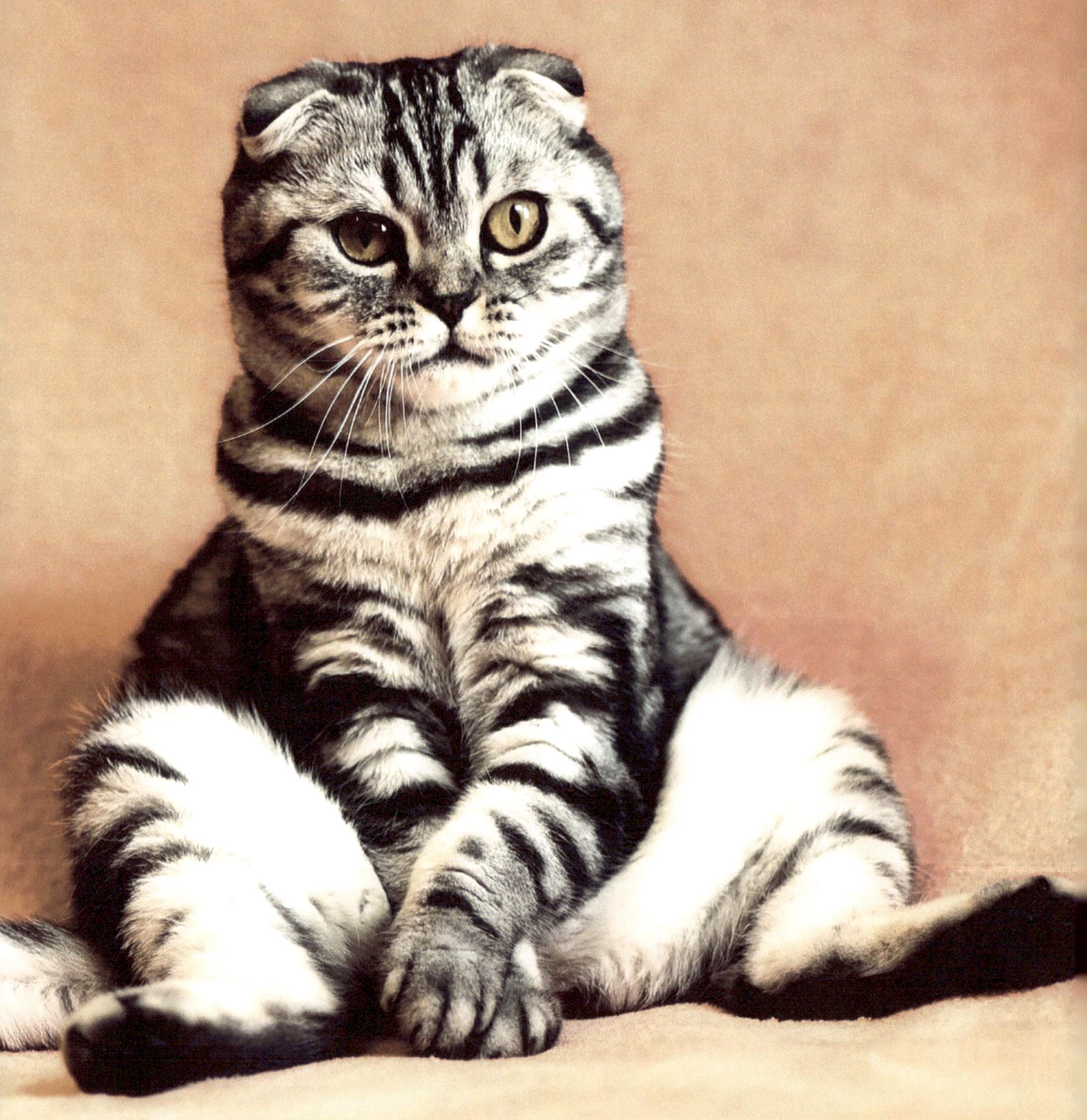

SCOTTISH FOLD

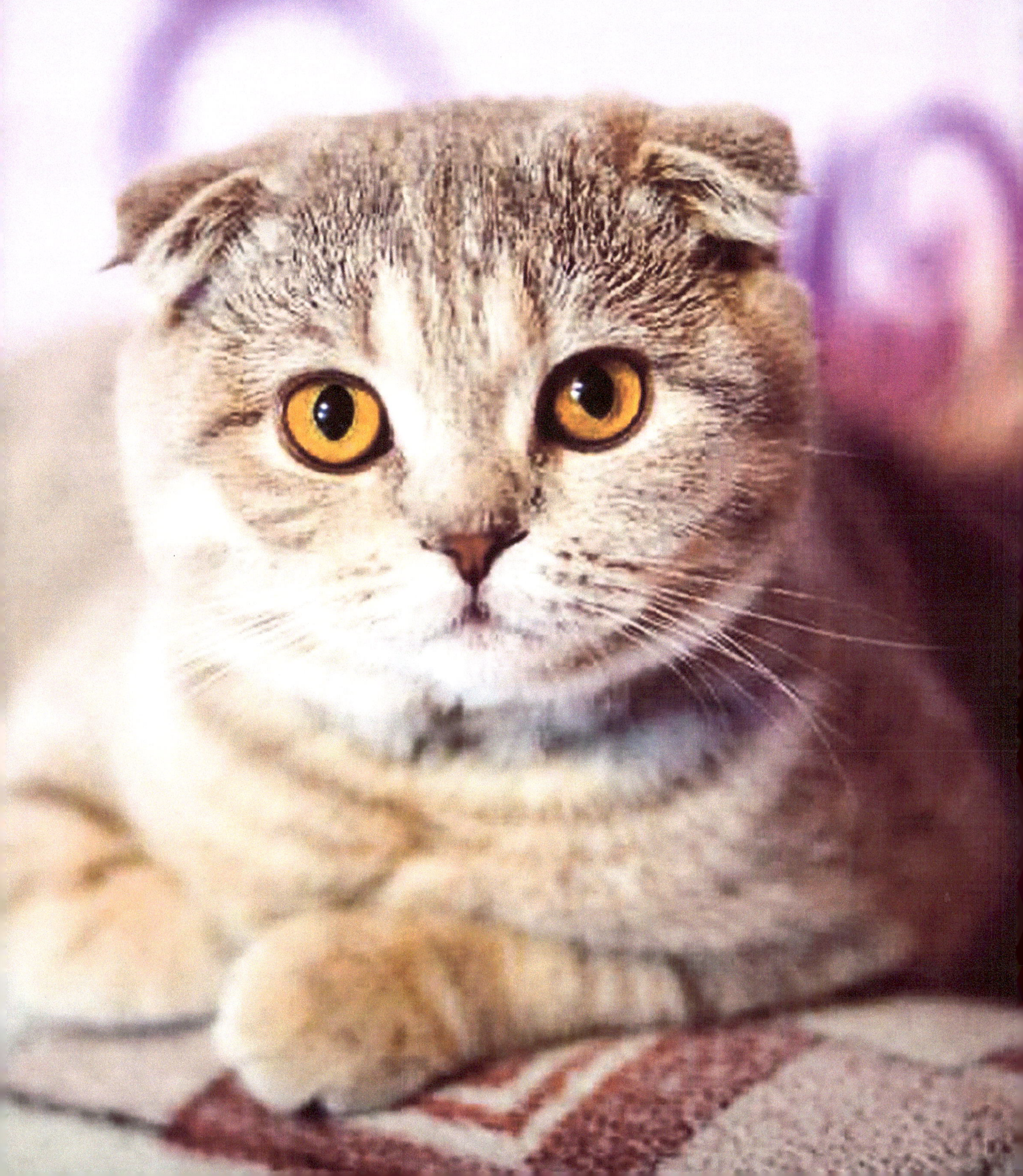

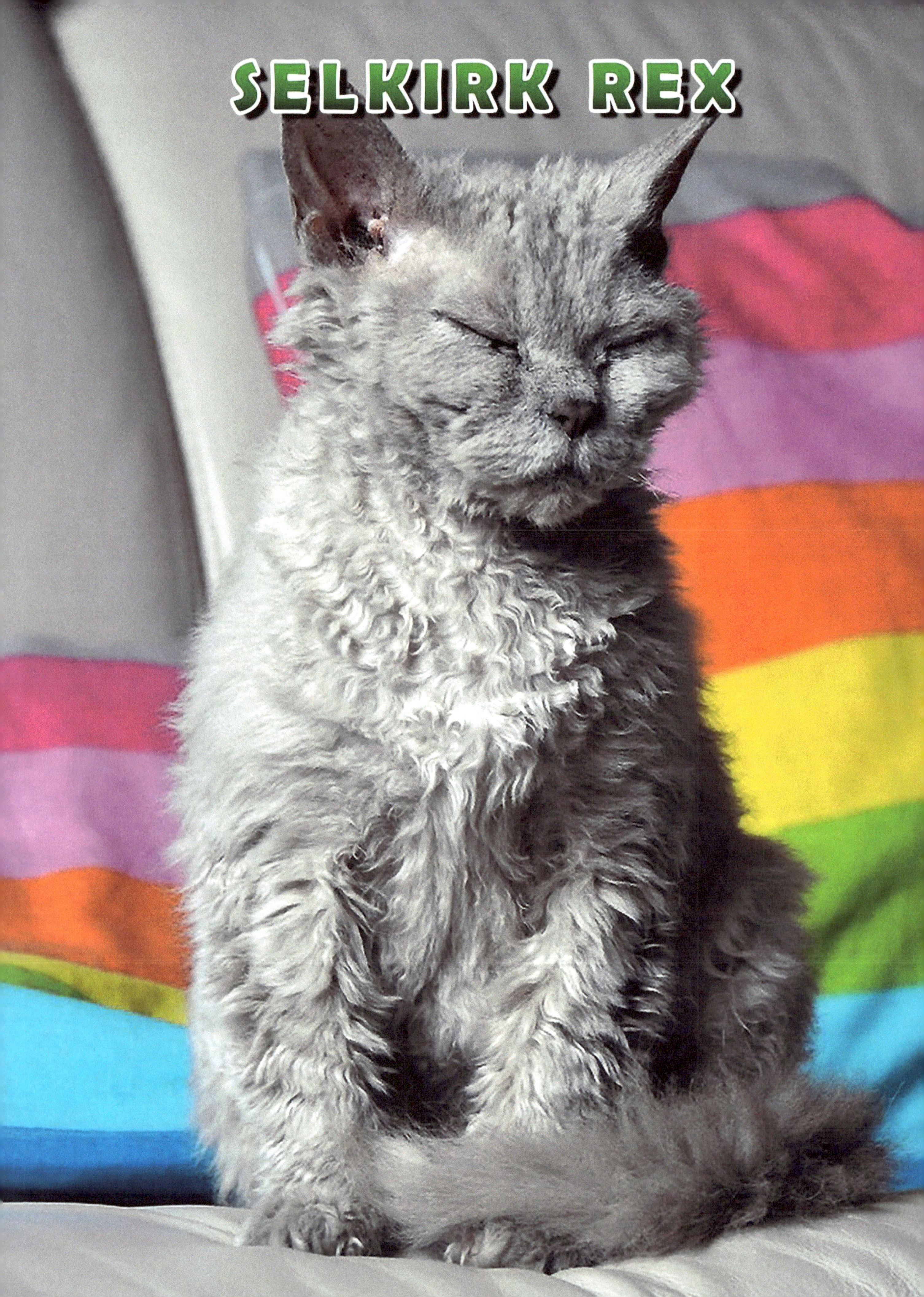
SELKIRK REX

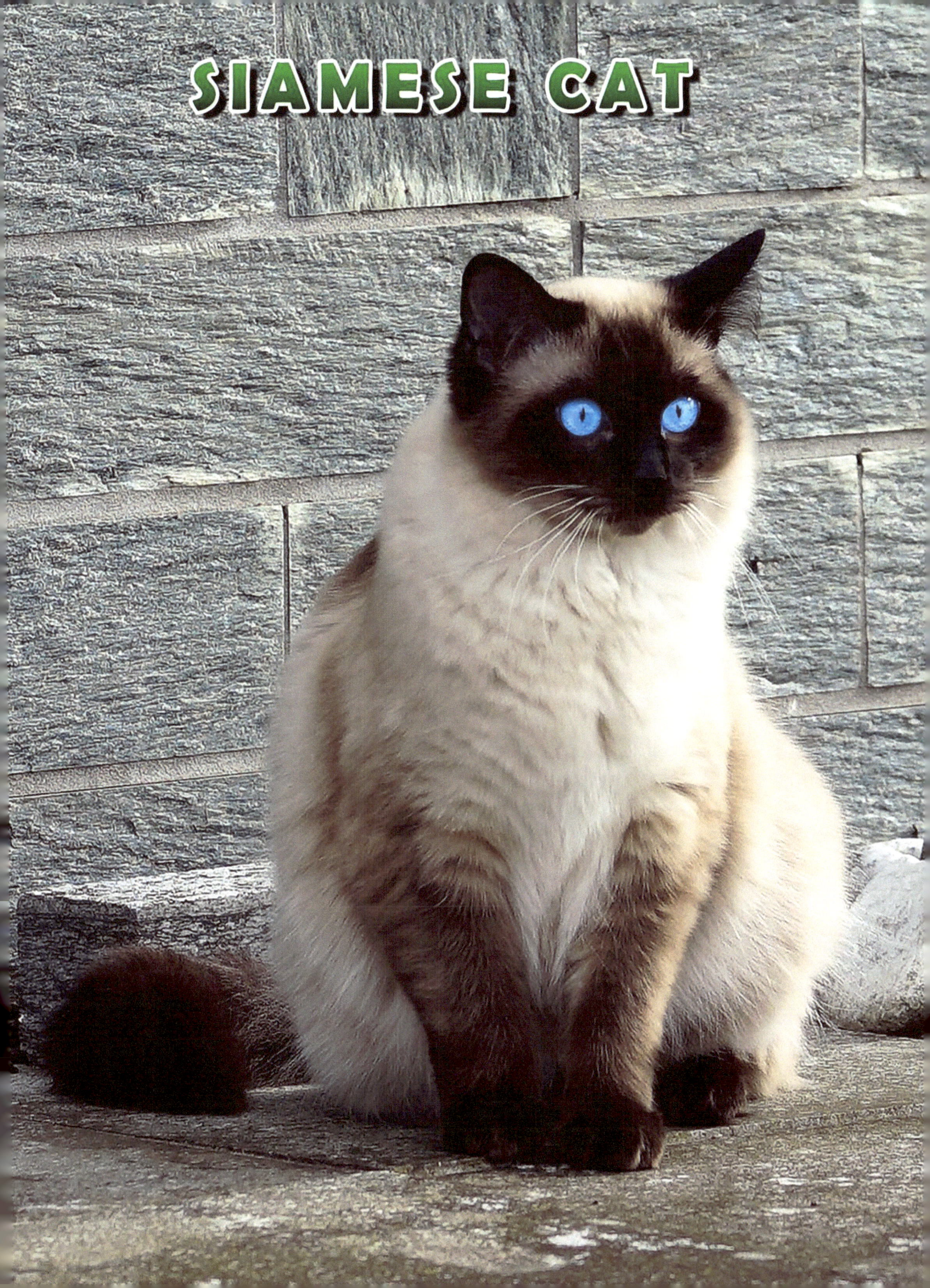
SIAMESE CAT

SIAMESE KITTEN

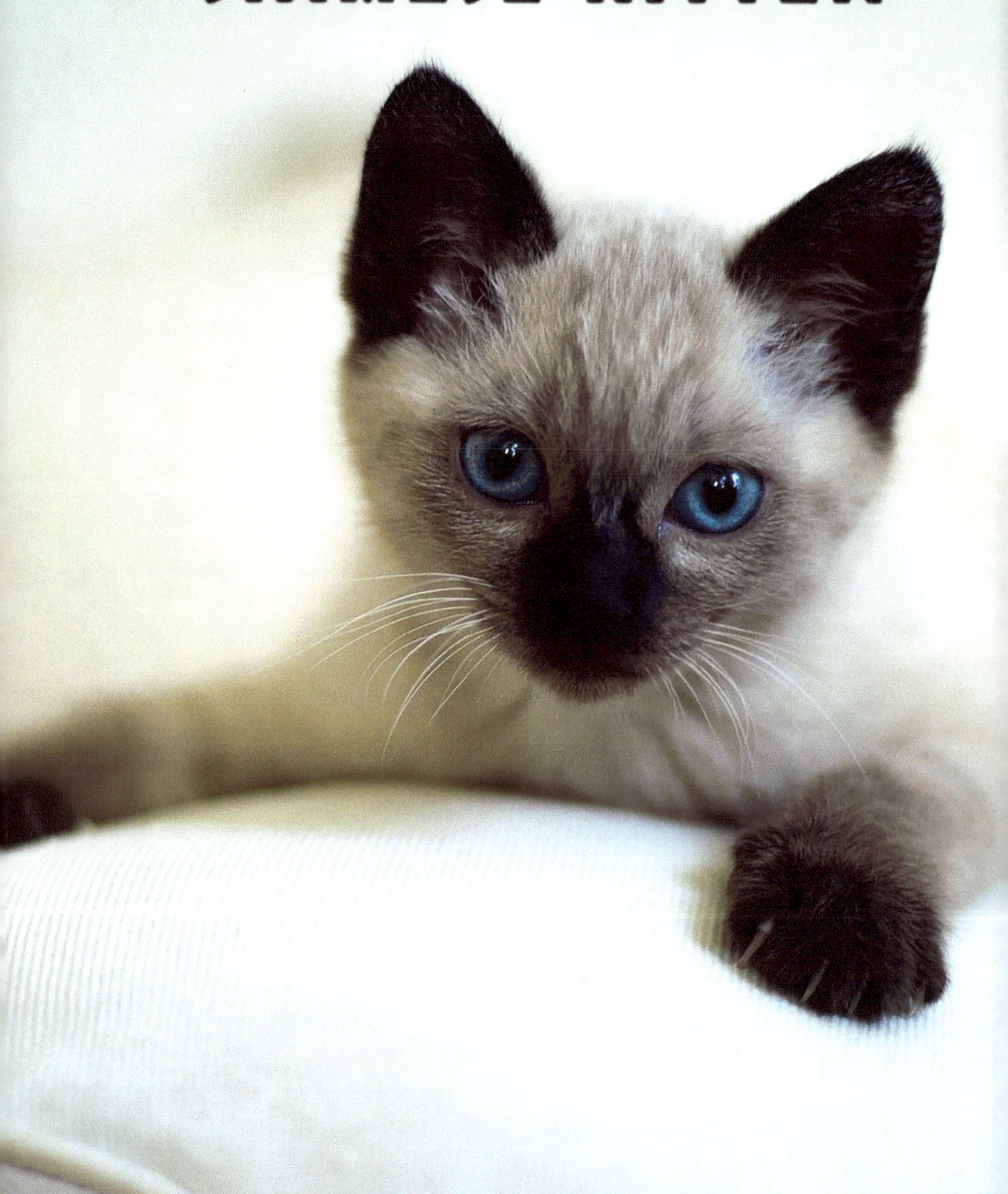

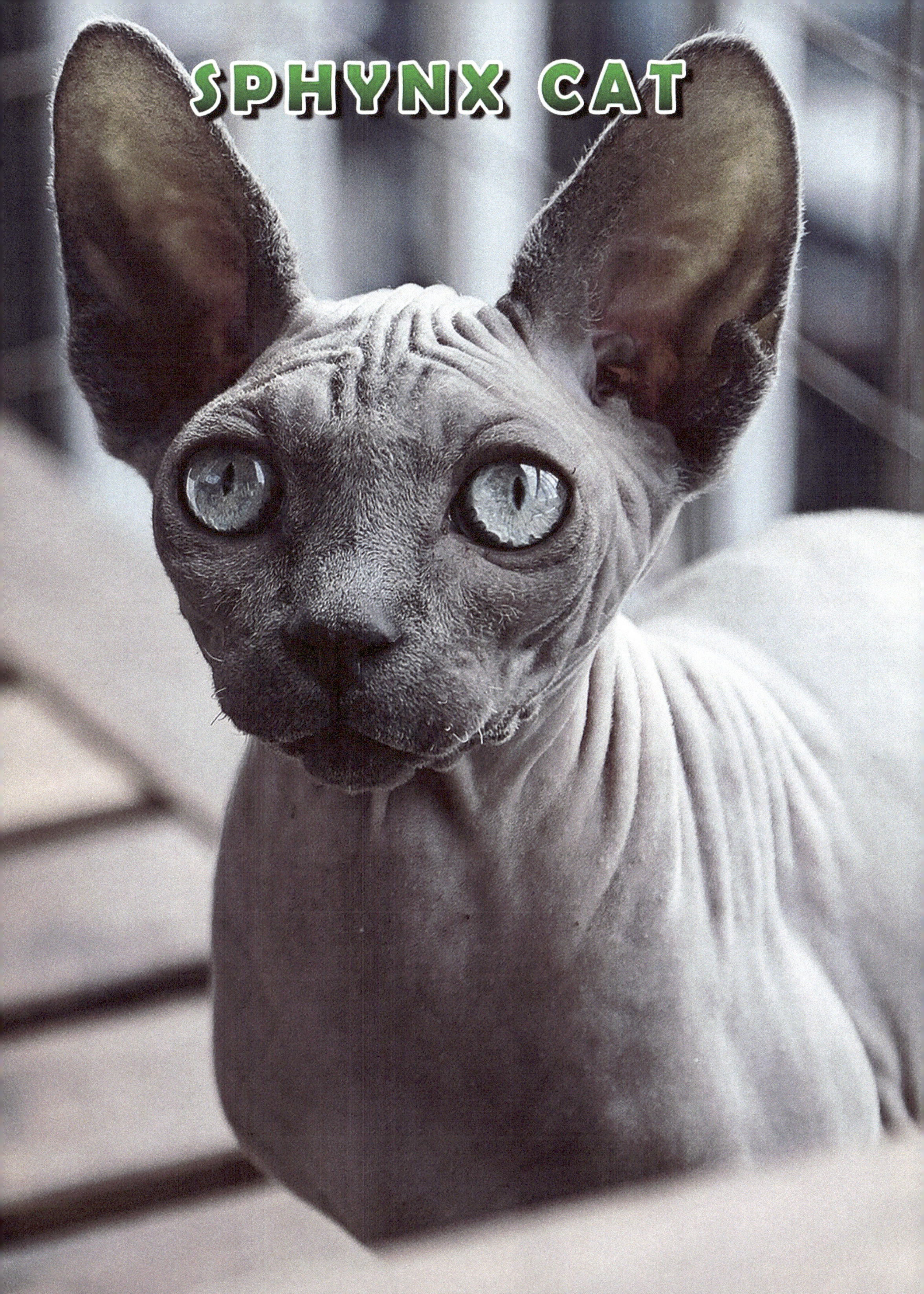
SPHYNX CAT

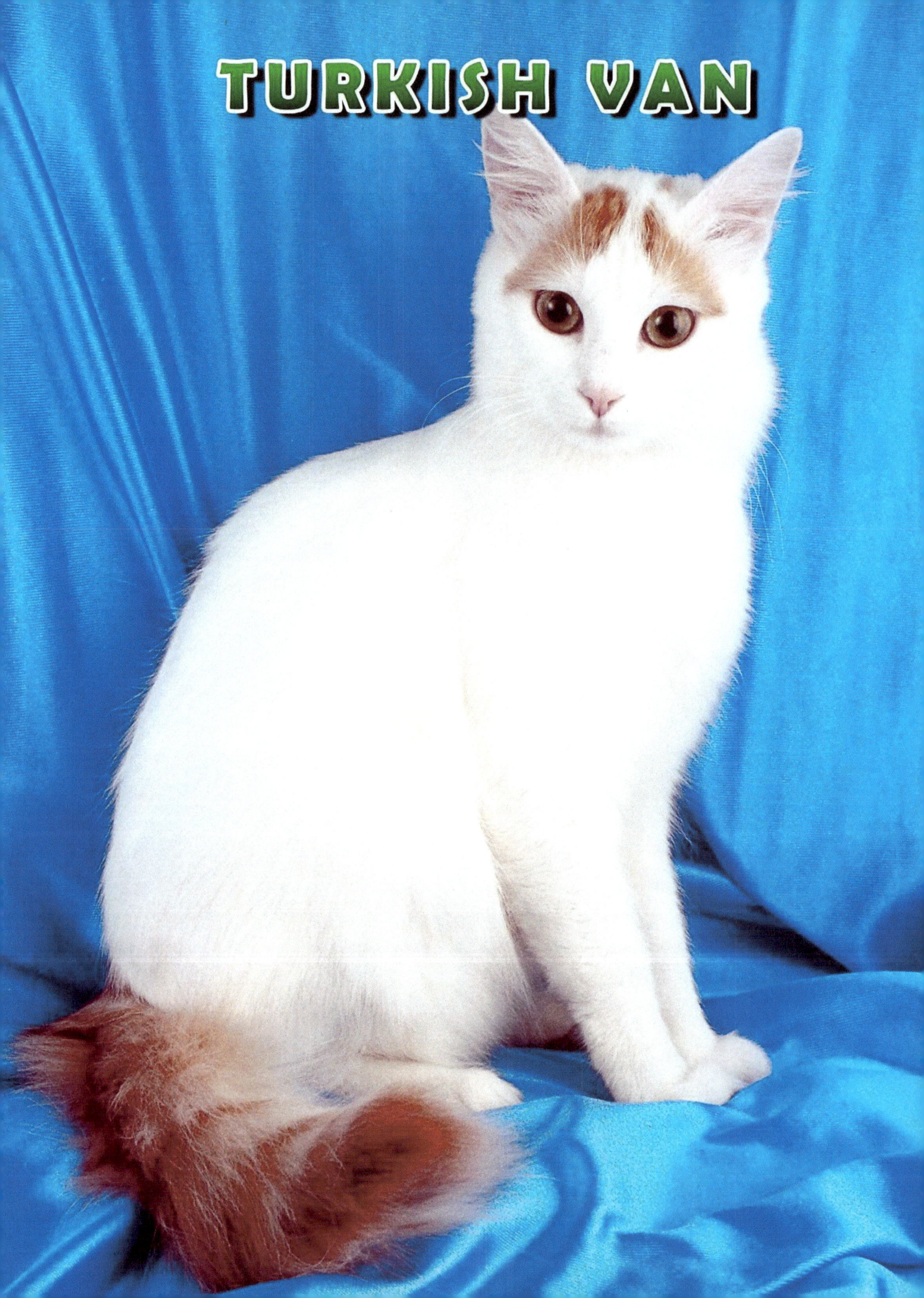
TURKISH VAN

TURKISH ANGORA

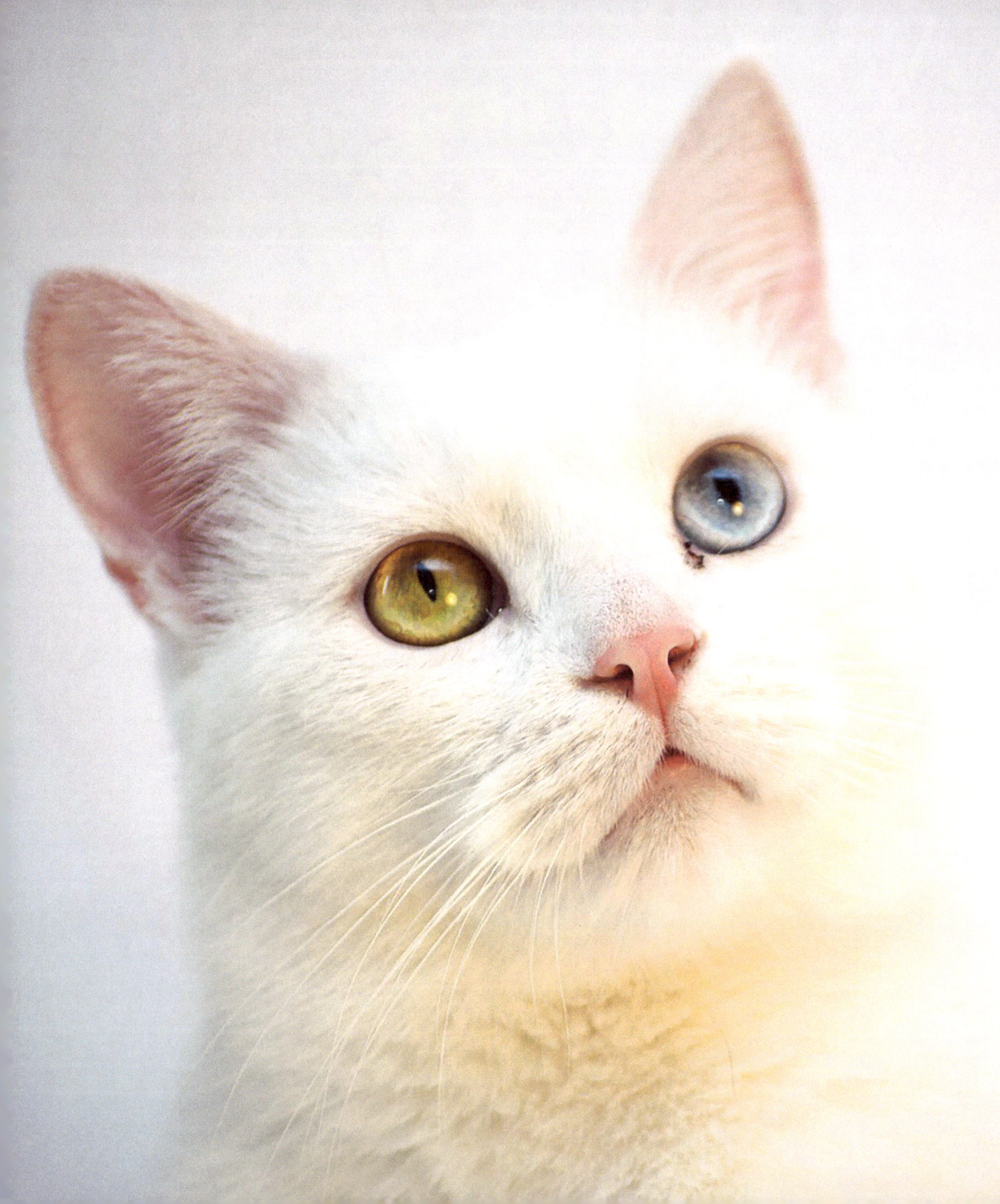

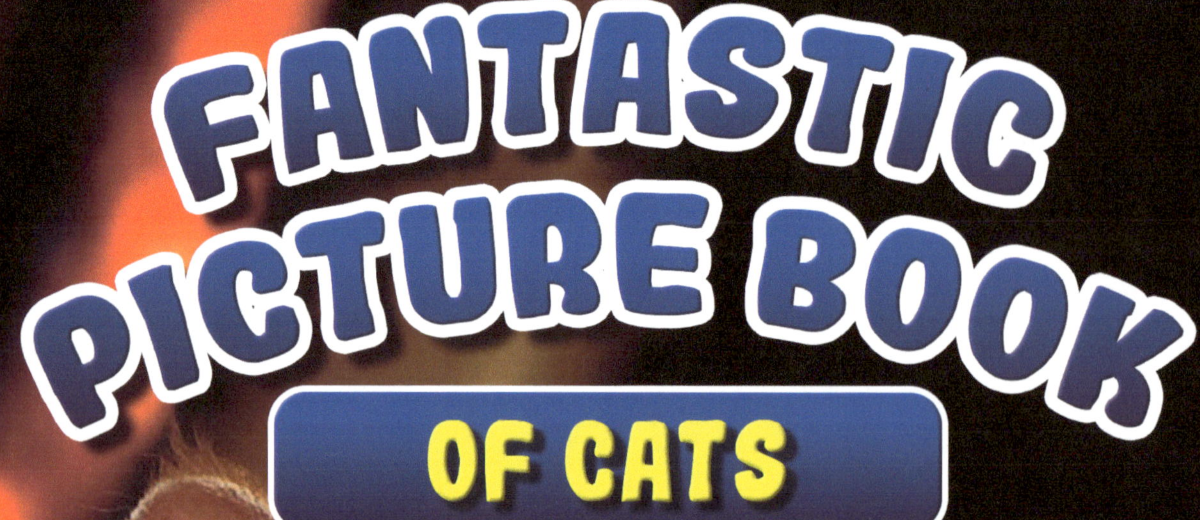

THANK YOU FOR PURCHASING THIS BOOK!

If you enjoyed it, please consider sharing it with your friends.

For more books, visit:
crypticfusion.com